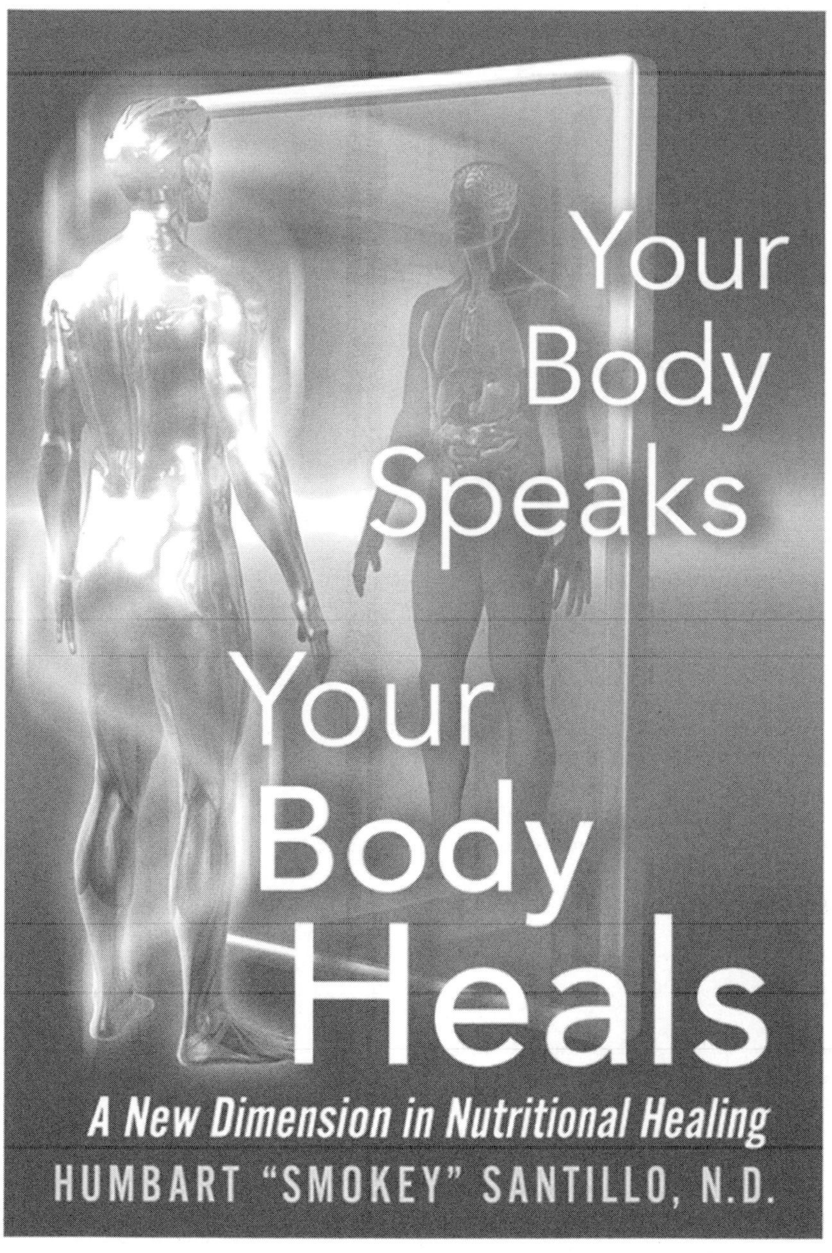

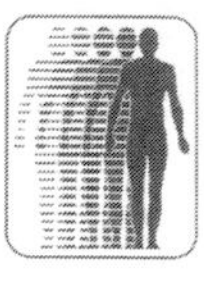

Designs for Wellness Press
Carlsbad, California © 2009

First Edition

ISBN: 978-0-9641952-7-1

Designs for Wellness Press
P.O. Box 1671
Carlsbad, CA 92018-1671
888-796-5229

Editors: Kate B. Johnson, B.A., and Roy E. Vartabedian, Dr.P.H.

The information in this book reflects the author's experience and current research. It is not intended to be used to replace or supersede individualized medical or professional advice. Before starting any nutrition or exercise program, you should consult a physician or other appropriate health professional to supervise your overall program.

Cover Illustration by Oliver Burston
www.DebutArt.com

Cover Design by George Foster
www.FosterCovers.com

Illustrations on pages 33, 43, and 68 by
Eric Lindley www.PartnersPhoto.com

Index by Madge Walls
www.AllSkyIndexing.com

Printed in the United States of America

Other publications by Dr. Santillo:

Herbal Combinations from Authoritative Sources
Natural Healing with Herbs
Natural Healing Herbal Correspondence Course
Intuitive Eating: Everybody's Guide to Lifelong Health and Vitality Through Food
The Basics of Intuitive Eating
Food Enzymes: The Missing Link to Radiant Health
ProMetabolics: Your Personal Guide to Transformational Health and Healing

---

Visit Dr. Santillo's Web site: **www.SmokeySantillo.com** **888-796-5229**
Volume discounts available.

Dedication

This book is dedicated to all of the Juice Plus+® distributors around the world. I would also like to thank Mike Barnhart, biologist, for his pristine efforts in research, development, and furthering the understanding of Juice Plus+® and its benefits. Your insight and dedication are honored and appreciated. Another big thank-you goes to Jeff Roberti, who had the vision and intuition about how an idea can manifest.

About the Author

Humbart "Smokey" Santillo, N.D.

Dr. Santillo is recognized as a visionary and pioneer in the growing field of Natural Therapeutics. He is the author of eight books—including the best-selling *Food Enzymes: The Missing Link to Radiant Health* and *Natural Healing with Herbs,* and his latest, *ProMetabolics: Your Personal Guide to Transformational Health and Healing*—read by more than 3.5 million people worldwide. A member of the Naturopathic Medical Association, he holds several patents in the field of nutrition and is highly sought after by sports shows and talk shows.

Born and raised in Lockport, New York, Dr. Santillo received a Bachelor of Science degree from Edinboro State Teacher's College in Pennsylvania, attending on football and track scholarships.

He subsequently developed 33 allergies and the early stages of rheumatoid arthritis; three years of suffering through traditional treatments with little or no relief launched his passionate, life-long quest for better health. Seeking answers and alternatives, he earned the degrees of Doctor of Naturopathy, Health Practitioner, and Master Herbalist. With his own health restored, he has since offered counseling and healing to more than 30,000 patients through his practice.

In 1995 at the U.S. Track and Field World Masters Games, comprising 6,400 athletes from 74 countries, Dr. Santillo anchored his 4 x 100-meter relay team to a gold medal victory. In the same year, he also broke two state records in the 100- and 200-meter races at the Empire State Games in New York, and won the Canadian Nationals in both the 100- and 200-meter races. He continues to compete today, recently taking first place in the 100-meter race at the 2008 New Jersey State Finals, and first place in the Tampa Bay "Beat the Heat" 100-Meter Masters race in May of 2009. At age 61 he competed and won in the 45 age category.

Table of Contents

Introduction

Your Body Speaks—Your Body Heals is a book written for the layperson and the health practitioner who are truly interested in assisting the body to heal itself. The wisdom of healing is within us; we simply have to learn how to support and release that healing power. An understanding of how to heal is the greatest gift we can give ourselves. We create most of our health problems, and learning how to *re-create* health is the main theme of this book. The fatigue and other symptoms that the body expresses are nothing more than physical and energetic imbalances speaking directly to us. This book explains how to read your body's language of symptoms and imbalances, and how to help bring it back into a healthy state. We must take control and be responsible for our own health.

This book synthesizes principles of Eastern and Western medicine into a simple method you can use to compound foods and herbs into formulas to support all functions of the body. Although we have been taught that any symptom or disease is a disturbance in one part of the body, this is incorrect, as the whole body is an energetic and physiological unit, in which every chemical and physical activity is interconnected. Whether there is one symptom or more, every bodily function is affected. Therefore, we must use a holistic approach to bring the entire bodily system back into a healing state. By a holistic approach, I mean any therapies, medical or nonmedical or both in combination, that bring the body back into balance. It makes no difference whether it's a common cold or cancer that the body is expressing—all organs and functions need to be supported. The foundational healing system in this book *does just that*.

Detoxification and nutritional support methods using foods, supplements, and herbs are the cornerstones of what I call the Triad Approach to healing. This approach supports all organs and functions in general and certain ones in particular, according to whatever disease (lack of ease) is present. It will give you the knowledge and confidence to heal yourself, or to support any therapy that is being administered. The layperson and doctor can learn and use this system easily. When it comes to healing, the patient cannot leave it up to the doctor, nor should the doctor leave it up to the patient; both must agree on a therapeutic approach and work together.

In no way does this system of healing take the place of a doctor or any specific therapy. Rather, it is a simple, integrated approach that everybody can use, a common ground. Whether you're a massage therapist, medical doctor, homeopath, nutritionist, or any other health practitioner, the method taught in this book is a foundational healing system that supports all other methods. A system like this should be used initially and during treatments, because if all bodily functions are not supported while treating a specific condition, other health problems can be created. An example would be going to a chiropractor and getting an adjustment, which releases energy to the heart or kidneys—doesn't it make sense, then, to provide your circulation, kidneys, and heart with good nutrition and maybe some herbal support? We can't always depend on the body to heal itself if the right materials (nutrients) are not present. And the body may be so damaged or toxic that without a systemic approach in support of healing, releasing energy in one part of the body will only create an imbalance in another. *Nature unaided can fail.*

How the body speaks and how the body heals are expressions of the warrior within. I hope this book will bring you peace and understanding, as well as a sense of the unity and interconnection of the body's functions, that you may fully appreciate these truths within us and between us.

To the wisdom within,

Dr. Humbart "Smokey" Santillo

Chapter 1
Environmental Causes of Disease

The body is wise; it heals itself. When this healing process is interfered with, the body becomes weaker, the immune system begins to fail, and sickness results. There is growing agreement that symptoms of what we call disease are primarily the result of toxicity, deficiencies, and imbalances in our lifestyle and environmental surroundings. However, it's very difficult for any health professional to convince his/her patients that the pain or disorder they are experiencing is caused by the food they're eating or the environment they live in.

Environmental factors—such as air pollution, water contamination, even electromagnetic fields in our homes—are hidden hazards, less talked about by physicians and the public simply because this information is not yet as widespread as dietary information. This doesn't mean it's less important, but many doctors don't have ways to diagnose and treat imbalances caused by environmental toxicity and electromagnetic forces. This chapter examines the hazards in our lives to get a clearer picture of what we're up against.

Electromagnetic Pollution

> Any new theory first is attacked as absurd, then admitted to be true, but obvious and insignificant. Finally, it seems to be important; so important that its adversaries claim that they themselves discovered it.
> —*William James*

Most people are not aware that they live in an electrical universe, surrounded by electro-vibratory fields that form and develop all physical bodies—nor do they realize that each of their own cells is an electrical universe in itself. The human body contains an estimated 200 quintillion cells (2 with 32 zeroes), so it encompasses a vast, invisible matrix of interrelating fields.

Cellular-electrical bodies. Each cell is made up of tiny electrical particles: protons, electrons, and others. Its nucleus holds tubular filaments—chromosomes and mitochondria—made of insulating materials and filled with a conducting fluid that contains the same mineral salts as sea water. The filaments are comparable to oscillating circuits, with the capacity to store energy and induce their own frequency and current.

Scientist George Lakhovsky postulated that the cell absorbs, emits, and radiates several frequencies. *(LaCabale Historire d'une De-couverte (L'oscillation Cellulaire), G. Dolw, Paris, 1934)* He realized that the cell works as a conductor, and that the energy flowing through it creates a unique electrical and magnetic field related to the cell's form and function. Lakhovsky further believed that all living cells wage a continual "war of radiations" against microbes; if the microbe's radiations "win," the cell ceases to oscillate at a healthy level and eventually dies.

It is important for our cellular-electrical bodies to vibrate at their appropriate frequencies. Richard Gerber's book *Vibrational Medicine (Bear and Company, Santa Fe, NM, 1988)* presents the body as a process of multidimensional energy systems that constantly interact in a harmonic fashion. If these systems become imbalanced, pathological symptoms can manifest on the physical, mental, and emotional planes. For the body to return to a higher level of health, its energy fields must be balanced and the sources of interference eliminated.

Scientists have many tools to observe the body's energies. An electrocardiogram (EKG) displays the heart's electrical activity. Electromyography (EMG) shows the flow of electricity along nerves. A polygraph simultaneously records the activity of the brain, skin, heart, respiratory system, and muscles. Biofeedback devices allow you to monitor and adjust your own brain waves, heart rate, temperature, blood flow and pressure, even digestive capabilities.

Electromagnetic fields. The sun, moon, planets—in fact, all living things and inorganic substances generate electromagnetic fields (EMFs), because everything consists of electrical particles. Natural EMFs surround us and move through us constantly.

The Earth and our physical bodies vibrate at roughly the same frequency, approximately 8 hertz.

But when we come into contact with artificially generated EMFs, we can become electrically imbalanced. Power lines, radio and microwave towers, radar, computers, video and television screens, radios, telephones, all electrical devices and appliances, cars, planes, motorcycles, and many other sources produce EMFs that interact with the membranes of living cells:

> We now live in a sea of electromagnetic radiation that we cannot sense, and that never before existed on this earth. ELF (electrical low frequency) electromagnetic fields vibrate about 30–100 hertz. If weaker than the earth's fields, it interferes with our bodies' biological cycles. Chronic stress and impaired disease resistance is the result. Recent studies of mice exposed for 30 days to 60-cycle electro-fields, whose strength was similar to those found near high-voltage transmission lines, revealed changes in hormone patterns, body weight, and blood chemistry, producing all the signs of chronic stress. But also, the study showed increase in degenerative disease, particularly those related to decreased competency of the immune system, such as cancer. *(Becker RO, Selden G. The Body Electric. William Morrow, NY, 1985)*

Health consequences. A striking example is the effect of introducing modern electrical communication systems to a rural area in Bavaria. The local people's health and longevity had been remarkable—until a mere six months after the installation of power lines and microwave towers for radio, telephones, and TV, when these healthy people began having heart attacks, cancer, and cavities, all previously unheard of. *(www.alternative-magnetic-therapy.com/emf-pollution.html)*

Video display terminals (VDTs) came under suspicion in the late 1970s for unexplained miscarriages, neonatal deaths, and birth defects in groups of women working with computers. A study of 1,583 pregnant California women in 1988 found that those who worked with VDTs 20 or more hours per week had an 80 percent greater chance of miscarrying than those who did similar work without VDTs. Another study linked high-current power lines and transformers to cancer in children; yet another found an unusually high percentage of electricians, electrical engineers, and utility repairmen in a group of 951 men who died of brain tumors. *(Goldhaber MK et al. The risk of miscarriage and birth defects among women who use visual display terminals during pregnancy. Am J Ind Med 1988 13:695–706; Lin RS et al. Occupational exposure to electromagnetic fields and the occurrence of brain tumors. An analysis of possible associations. J Occup Med 1985 27:413–419; Wertheimer N, Leeper E. Electrical wiring configurations and childhood cancer. Am J Epidemiol 1979 109:273–284)*

Our homes and workplaces are filled with electrical wiring, devices, and machines that create their own EMFs. These unnatural energies, especially those produced by alternating 60-cycle current, are suspected causal factors in depression, suicide, cancer, leukemia, psychosis, cataracts—and the list grows daily. For detailed information on this subject, I suggest Robert Becker's book *Cross Currents: The Perils of Electro-Pollution (Jeremy P. Tarcher, Los Angeles, CA, 1990).*

Electromagnetic pollution solutions. One way to protect yourself from some electromagnetic pollution is to use polarizers that absorb, concentrate, and radiate a broad spectrum of wavelengths. Life Field Polarizers, in small portable versions and larger sizes for the home or office, are available from Internet suppliers. Another way is to wear a Teslar watch, intended to shield the wearer against extra-low frequencies (ELFs) by putting out a constant 8-hertz scalar wave (available from Teslar Global Technologies, www.teslartech.com).

The Air We Breathe

Each human being breathes 15,000–20,000 liters of air per day. Meanwhile, millions of pounds of toxic chemicals are routinely emitted into that air each year. Pollutants from power plants, factories, incinerators, and automobiles have turned our skies, lakes, and rivers into toxic dumps. These toxins kill trees, plants (including crops), insects, birds, fish, and other wildlife. They have altered the weather patterns and destroyed the earth's protective barrier against harmful rays, and they threaten virtually all living organisms on this planet.

Health consequences. It is estimated that 1,700 cancers per year in the United States are caused by airborne emissions. This figure does not reflect the other health effects of these hundreds of chemicals that have been identified as causing birth defects, sterility, neurological disorders, kidney or liver damage, headaches, nausea, rashes, respiratory diseases, eye, nose, and throat problems, and more.

In many US cities, because of dangerously high ozone levels due to air pollution, people are occasionally warned against exercising outdoors, and pregnant women or people older than 60 are cautioned against going out at all. The day may not be too far off when children walk to school with ultraviolet protectors and respirators.

Inadequate regulation. Air pollution is the least-regulated of toxic releases. Federal and state laws have focused mainly on water and land pollution. The federal Clean Air Act has not been strong enough over the last 19 years, with EPA emission standards set for few of the 70,000 toxic chemicals in use.

In 1988, the Emergency Planning and Community Right-to-Know Act (Title III of the Super Fund Amendment and Restoration Act) required major industries to disclose information on the toxic chemicals they release into our air, water, sewage systems and treatment plants, and landfill areas. Unfortunately, this act has major limitations; for example, the information disclosure it requires is based on the industry's own estimates, with no governmental verification.

According to the information provided by industries in New York State alone, 87,000,000 pounds of toxins were reportedly released into the air. Forty percent came from cracks in valves, pipes, open chemical tanks, and the like—and was, therefore, unregulated! The other 60 percent came from industrial smokestacks. And only 683 of New York's 14,500 industrial plants submitted information for inclusion in that report.

Hazards of indoor air. Indoor air pollution is a major cause of disease but an area of widespread ignorance. Fact: the average person spends about 90 percent of his/her time indoors. Fact: 80 percent of building materials are artificial products incorporating concrete, plastics, steel, aluminum, and more, chemically treated or coated with toxic paint. Molecules of all of these materials make their way into the air. Of the many thousands of chemicals currently in use, some are already known to cause cancer and mutagenic diseases, as well as allergies, asthma, dermatitis, headaches, and fatigue. There are even health conditions called Sick Building Syndrome (SBS) and Building-Related Disease (BRD). Annually, 500,000 workdays are lost because of sickness from these poisons in the air.

Consider the example of wall-to-wall carpets. Almost all carpets are made of synthetic fibers derived from petroleum, which is bad enough. But they're also treated with stain-resistant or fire-resistant chemicals, and then most likely saturated with fungicides and pesticides too. Once laid on the floor, a carpet emits powerful fumes. These chemicals cause allergies, headaches, and malformed cells. As a carpet gets old, it emits dust and fibers that circulate through the building's heating system, which causes sinus and respiratory problems for many people—and shampooing or steam-cleaning carpets can actually aggravate health conditions by adding even more chemicals to the indoor air.

Additional household toxins are found in bleach, fabric softener, spray starch, children's sleepwear, mothballs, insect spray, pesticide, scented toilet paper, toothpaste, cosmetics, shampoo, aluminum cookware, tobacco smoke, fireplaces, and much more—even supermarket-sold milk and produce.

Due to their small size and faster respiratory rates, children are particularly vulnerable to health problems from both indoor and outdoor toxins. Most building air pollutants are heavier than air, so they hang lower, closer to a child's nose and mouth. Children's bodies are also not fully equipped to process toxins, increasing their health risks. Many household poisons are accidentally ingested, splashed in the eyes, absorbed through the skin, or inhaled—and of the five to ten million household poisonings reported annually, most of the victims are children.

Indoor pollution solutions. Unfortunately, when we read about toxins in our lives, we often throw up our hands, feel defeated, and do nothing about it. But this only allows things to get worse—not only for us, but for everybody's children. We must all start doing something. Simply by using air purifiers and water filtration systems, you can help prevent major health disorders for yourself and your family. I suggest Deborah Lynn Dadd's terrific and informative book, *The Non-Toxic Home (Jeremy P. Tarcher, Los Angeles, CA, 1986),* which gives plenty of suggestions on how to create and live in a safe indoor environment.

PESTICIDES FOUND IN GROUNDWATER ACCORDING TO THE EPA

ORIGINAL LIST: 20 PESTICIDES

Alachlor
Aldricarb (sulfoxide and sulfton)
Atrazinde
Bromacil
Carbfuran
Cyanazine
DBCP
ACPA (and acid products)
Dicamba
1,2-Dichloropropane
Dinoseb
EDB
Fonofos
Metolachlor
Metribuzin
Oxamyl
Propachlor
Symazine
Terbufos
1,2,3-Trichloropropane

NEW LIST: ANOTHER 43 PESTICIDES

Aldrin
Ametryn
Alpha-BHC
Atratone
Gamma-BHC
Cabaryl
Chloropyrifos
Chlordane
Chlorothalonil
DDD
DDE (degradent of DDT)
DDT
Dacthal
Diazinon
Dieldrin
Disyston
ETU (degradent of Maneb)
EBDCs
Endosulfan endrin
Heptachlor hexazinone
Isofenfos
Lindane
Linuron
MCPA
Malathion
Metalaxyl
Methyl parathuion
Para-nitrophenol
Paraquat
Parathion
Pentachlorophenol
Picloram
Propazine
Silvex
Sulprofos
TCP (degradent of Trychlopyr)
Toxaphene
Trifluralin
1,3-Dichloropropene
2,4-D
2,4,5-T
2,6-Dichlobenzoic acid

Fighting Air and Water Pollution

The Right-to-Know Act is a powerful tool that we can use to protect the environment and ourselves by learning about emissions and demanding tougher laws and safer practices. Industries aren't required to provide toxic release information directly to the public, but the Department of Environmental Conservation (DEC) and local Emergency Planning Committees are mandated to provide this information. To request it, you can write to USEPA, Attention: Public Inquiry, P.O. Box 70266, Washington, DC 20024-0266; or, you can call the EPA Right-to-Know Hotline at 800-535-0202.

Once you're informed, educate your community. Build cases against companies to reduce their emissions. You can request that a company test around its site for toxins; if they refuse, call the DEC and request testing of the groundwater, soil, and air emissions. You can investigate the companies in your area to see which ones have reduced their toxic emissions. Then make public statements via radio, television, or newspaper, asking why other companies haven't followed suit. Good luck!

Chapter 2
Detoxification: The First Step

Note: If you're nervous or unsure about undertaking a cleansing diet or detoxification, see a physician or health practitioner who specializes in these matters. Usually there's no problem, but it's better to be safe than sorry.

The "worker within" knows the difference between high- and low-quality food. When you start improving your diet, an amazing thing happens. Every cell immediately begins to use the good stuff and to discard any remnants from the past, eliminating residues and waste products from the low-quality food and other harmful substances you've taken in: meat, eggs, cheese, preservatives, drugs, caffeine, nicotine, and more. After getting rid of the gunk and the junk, your body can rebuild itself from the healthful nutrients you're giving it.

If the body could talk, it would say, "Look at all this great raw food and fresh juice. Let's get rid of all the old bile in the gallbladder, clean the liver, the blood, the joints, the veins, the capillaries. Let's clean out all the old debris, so we can rebuild everything with this fresh, live material."

The scientific term for that inner housecleaning and breaking-down process is catabolism. When the body begins to burn or eliminate the waste, you might experience a fever, or get drippy sinuses, or diarrhea, or a rash. Symptoms that you experienced recently or even years ago may reoccur. This is all a natural part of catabolism. When the catabolic phase passes in three to ten days, the symptoms disappear.

Next, anabolism begins, a renewing, building-up process. The anabolic phase is your reward, and you may feel wonderful—but it won't last long, because as soon as the body builds up its strength, it can start self-cleansing again. After all, it's impossible to get rid of years of accumulated poisons in only three to ten days; that would overburden the eliminatory organs and could even cause severe degenerative problems.

So the cycle of phases continues as the body gradually becomes cleaner, stronger, and healthier. I call this "the cyclic nature of health transitions." Keep in mind that not everybody experiences adverse symptoms when the body is cleansing itself, and most inconveniences from these symptoms are slight.

The Healing Crisis

A healing crisis is defined in naturopathy as "an acute reaction, resulting from the activity of nature's healing forces in overcoming chronic disease conditions," but is acknowledged by few doctors in the conventional allopathic tradition. It is brought about when the body becomes overloaded with waste and poisons. The tissues begin to throw out these unwanted substances, which are carried by the bloodstream to the eliminatory organs: the bowels, kidneys, lungs, skin, nasal passages, ears, throat, and genito-urinary tract. As a result, these organs can become irritated and congested, leading to symptoms such as colds, itching, boils, sores, kidney and bladder infections, perspiration, diarrhea, and fever.

A process of elimination. These symptoms are part of the cure. There's nothing to fear—but you must work *with* them. *Do not* suppress them with drugs unless absolutely necessary; our organs weren't nature-made to handle such chemicals, so drugs accumulate in fatty tissue and other parts of the body, and tissues imbedded with these foreign elements begin to degenerate. (Many natural healers claim certain diseases are actually "drug diseases"—that is, caused by these inimical elements, which suppress nature's healing forces.)

The characteristics and duration of a healing crisis depend largely upon the following factors:

1. **Waste/toxin type.** Excess mucus forced out through the mucous membranes often produces nasal drip and other characteristic cold-and-flu symptoms. Elimination of drugs, uric acid, and other substances may manifest in different ways.

2. **Condition of eliminatory organs.** If waste/toxin elimination through the usual pathways is inadequate, the body may burn them off (fever) or store them (e.g., boils or acne). During a healing crisis, pain in the kidneys, bladder, or bowels might lead you to believe that the painful organ is malfunctioning or diseased—but in fact, it's more likely your strongest or best-adapted eliminatory organ and is very busy as a primary outlet.
3. **Energy level or vitality.** A robust person eliminates waste/toxins more quickly; elimination takes longer for a weak body with low vitality, especially if you've been ill.
4. **Area of waste/toxin congestion.** If it's the lungs, this can manifest as respiratory symptoms; if it's the bowel, constipation and then diarrhea can occur.
5. **Climate/weather.** During hot weather, with lighter clothing and more exposure to the sun, more of your waste/toxin load can be drawn to the surface and thrown out through the skin. During cold weather, the skin is usually covered, so the body must make extra use of the kidneys, bowel, and lungs for elimination.

Warning signs. A healing crisis can often be avoided if you have a strong constitution and properly functioning eliminatory organs. Sometimes a "preview" of a major elimination indicates an oncoming crisis—watch for dark urine, fever, headache, ringing in the ears, coated tongue, irritability, weakness, and sluggishness. In this early stage, assistance from foods, herbs, enemas, homeopathy, acupuncture, massage, and hydrotherapy can often release energy blocked by accumulated waste and poisons, normalizing energy flow to the organs and facilitating elimination without a noticeable crisis. The crisis can't always be avoided, but these natural therapies always assist in restoring health and balance. Energy flow is discussed in chapter 3.

Healing crisis versus "disease crisis." Although these often look alike in their outward manifestations, they occur under different conditions in the body and have different results. Both begin when the overloaded body initiates an acute elimination reaction. If the body's healing forces are on the offensive or "ascending," a healing crisis develops. But if the body's on the defensive, a disease crisis develops—and if waste/toxins are not fully eliminated, the body adapts itself to them, stores them, and functions at a lower energy level. Waste/toxins continue to accumulate, inhibiting the organs' proper performance of their normal functions, and finally a chronic condition manifests.

It's important to differentiate between a healing crisis and a disease process. Any crisis that isn't monitored, understood, and properly treated can weaken the body and last longer than it should. If it's a healing crisis, there's usually a positive change after three days: the most severe symptoms lessen, fever breaks, and you become more relaxed and feel better. If after three days, however, the severe symptoms don't lessen, a new approach is indicated. *Note:* Consult a physician with any questions about the length or severity of a symptom, crisis, or illness.

Treatment and recovery. The use of foods, juices, and herbs for handling the symptoms of a crisis—or of a planned detoxification—is described in the next section. Once a crisis is over, whether you're weak or strong, toning and strengthening the body with exercise, proper diet, herbs, and hydrotherapy is a necessity. For information about how to do this, see my book *Natural Healing with Herbs (Hohm Press, Prescott, AZ, 1984).*

As natural living and a balanced diet support and strengthen the body, it automatically draws chronic waste from the tissues for regular elimination, and becomes stronger after each healing crisis. Crises occur less frequently, until the day comes when only health is present and sickness is history. You may still experience slight crises once in a while, but they'll usually be very brief (one to three days).

Detox: The Purification Diet for Inner Cleanliness

The purification diet's purpose is to cleanse the body. It's typically used for six to 14 days but can be extended if desired. In detoxification, it's better to take it slow than to rush it—trying to get "too pure too fast" can be destructive and postpone the achievement of your goal. Usually, a person who's been eating meat and processed foods should start with a six-day purification diet, whereas a vegetarian or a person who's been on cleansing diets before can stay on it longer. This diet can be used in full as often as every six to ten weeks.

A healing crisis is a normal part of the detox process. If adverse symptoms persist over a three- to six-day period, it usually means the body is extremely toxic; in such a case, I suggest alternating purification diet periods with periods of progressive changes in the regular diet. A good maintenance regime is a three-day purification diet at the end of every month, while improving your diet between cleanses.

Note: Sometimes cleansing diets and detox therapies don't work—chiefly, because organs overloaded with years of stored gunk become weak, and the body becomes fatigued, greatly prolonging the cleansing effort. For someone who hasn't been ill or worn down, the body has the endurance to tolerate cleansing herbs, fasting, and advanced water treatments. For someone who's weaker, energy-building foods, short fasts, and tonic herbs are commonly recommended; then, once the body's energy returns, more vigorous cleansing methods can be used.

During the Purification Diet...

You'll support your body during this diet with plenty of juices, and if necessary, with herbs. You want to assist detoxification and not to put excessive stress on the organs involved. So during the purification diet—or any cleansing diet—I strongly suggest the following:

- **Avoid stimulants and sedatives.** No caffeine is allowed. You should not ingest anything that would cause a stimulating or sedating reaction—you want to experience your body the way it really is.
- **Rest as much as possible.** If you feel well enough, you can do some light exercise such as walking.
- **Honor your individual needs.** If the diet's recommended

food is too much for you to eat, or if you are simply not hungry, skip a meal. If you do skip a meal, substitute for it with 2 cups of freshly made fruit or vegetable juice.

- **Take a probiotic supplement to support the bowel.** You can get these at your health food store; make sure the product contains bifidus and/or acidophilus cultures. Probiotics are discussed in chapter 3.
- **Take supplemental digestive enzymes before each meal.** Choose a product that contains the four major digestive enzyme groups: amylase, protease, lipase, and cellulase. Enzymes are discussed in chapter 3.

Using Juices for Detoxification and Organ Support

Freshly made fruit and vegetable juices help neutralize toxins and aid elimination through the kidneys and liver. Here are my recommendations for juice use to detoxify and support the body during this or any cleansing diet:

- **Dilution.** If you aren't accustomed to drinking juice, dilute it with 25 percent distilled, purified water, or water that's gone through a reverse-osmosis unit.
- **Dosage.** Drink 8–10 ounces of juice (or watered-down juice) at a time, a *minimum* of three times a day, between meals: a half-hour before meals, or one and a half hours after. Juice taken on an empty stomach is absorbed into the bloodstream *very* rapidly, usually in 5–15 minutes.
- **Type and timing.** I suggest fruit juices in the morning and during the day, and vegetable juices during the day and in the evening. Avoid fruit juices after 7:00 p.m., because their stimulating sugars may disturb your sleep.
- **Chewing.** Chew the pulp in your juice before swallowing; this is especially important if you have any symptoms of diabetes or hypoglycemia.
- **Side effects.** If the juices cause gas or bloating, reduce the amount you drink. If it becomes a real problem, omit them entirely; you can substitute vegetable broth or water. If gas or bloating continues, an enema should help.

Liquid chlorophyll, the juice of green plants, is one of the best blood-purifiers and nutritional supplements. For a tonic, drink 2 ounces of chlorophyll mixed with 4–6 ounces of apple, pineapple, or your favorite vegetable juice twice daily.

During your detox, choose juices that support any particular organ or system that you know to have a weakness. The chart below shows organ-specific juice combinations. If you can't find all the vegetables and fruits suggested, just use some of them.

JUICE COMBINATIONS

LIVER	CARROT, APPLE, AND DANDELION GREEN
KIDNEYS	CARROT, PARSLEY, AND APPLE
SKIN	BEET *(with beet top)*, CELERY, CUCUMBER, 1/4 POTATO, CARROT, AND APPLE
BLOOD	KALE, PARSLEY, GINGER *(small piece)*, APPLE, AND CARROT
BOWEL	SPINACH, APPLE, AND CARROT
GAS	CABBAGE, CARROT, AND APPLE
LUNGS	CARROT, PARSLEY, 1/4 POTATO, WATERCRESS, GINGER *(small piece)*, AND MUSTARD GREEN
ADRENALS	BEET *(with beet top)*, CELERY, AND ROMAINE
STOMACH	FENNEL, CABBAGE, CELERY, AND APPLE
BLADDER	ALL MELONS *(drink melon juice only by itself)* CARROT, BEET *(with beet top)*, CUCUMBER, AND PARSLEY
GALL-BLADDER	PARSLEY, BEET *(with beet top)*, APPLE, AND CELERY

Creating juice formulas for organ support is discussed further in chapter 3. I also recommend J. Kordich's *The Juiceman's Power of Juicing (William Morrow, NY, 1992).* He's been juicing for more than 40 years, and his book gives dozens of combinations for specific and general use.

Using Herbs for Detoxification, Organ Support, and Symptoms

If you've done a detox or cleansing diet before, then usually the diet—with plenty of liquids—is all you'll need. But if you wish, you can also use herbs to help purify the blood, or for additional support of weakened organs, or to relieve symptoms of a healing crisis. For example, if you have lower back pain possibly related to the kidneys, you could take an infusion of corn silk or juniper berry. If you become constipated, suggested herbal laxatives are turkey rhubarb, *Cascara sagrada,* or cold senna tea with a little ginger. A list of specific herbs for organs and symptoms is provided in chapter 3.

Many herbs are available as a convenient liquid extract called a tincture, usually taken as 25 drops to 1 cup of water three times a day, though doses vary. Some herbs are used as an infusion—basically, a strong tea. To make an infusion, put 1 ounce of the herb in a kettle or pot and add 1 pint of boiling water; cover and let steep for 20 minutes; strain out the herbs, and you have approximately 3 cups of infusion. The usual dose is 1 cup three times a day. (During a cleanse, you may wish to add juice to your infusions.) For an herb in capsule form—some are too bitter to take otherwise—the usual dose is two capsules three times a day. But during acute symptoms, any of these forms of herb are usually taken every two hours.

You can find herbal products at your local health food store. Herb companies I recommend include Nature's Way, Herb Pharm, and Gaia Herbs (www.naturesway.com, www.herb-pharm.com, and www.gaiaherbs.com).

The Purification Diet

Before Breakfast

- **Psyllium drink.** A half-hour before breakfast, mix 1 heaping teaspoon of psyllium seed powder in 8 ounces of orange, pineapple, or apple juice (use fresh juice when possible). Drink immediately before it thickens. Psyllium seed powder may cause bloating; for discomfort, use an enema or an herbal laxative for a few days.

Breakfast

- **Fresh, raw fruit.** Eat at least a half-pound of one fruit, or a salad of two to four fruits, from this list (organic and in season whenever possible): apple, apricot, berries, cherry, currant, fig, grape, grapefruit, guava, mango, melon nectarine, orange, papaya, peach, pear, persimmon, plum, ripe pineapple, and more. Melons should be eaten by themselves, *not* mixed with other fruits. While on this diet or any other detox regime, do *not* eat banana or avocado, because they slow detoxification and elimination.
- **Dried fruit.** You can also include organic, unsulphured dried fruits: apple, apricot, berries, cherry, currant, date, fig, mango, papaya, peach, pear, prune, pineapple, and raisin. *These must always be soaked to reconstitute*—if they're eaten dry, they'll cause fermentation in the intestinal tract.
- **No coffee, tea, milk, or other beverages.** For best digestion, do not drink any liquid with meals.

Before Lunch

- **Psyllium drink.** A half-hour before lunch, drink 1 heaping teaspoon of psyllium seed powder mixed in 8 ounces of orange, pineapple, or apple juice.

Lunch

- **Fresh, raw vegetables.** Eat a chopped salad of up to four of the vegetables from this list (organic and in season whenever possible): artichoke, asparagus, beet, Brussels

sprout, carrot, cauliflower, fresh corn, cucumber, celery, dandelion green, endive, eggplant, green bean, green pepper, kale, kohlrabi, lettuce (not iceberg), lotus, okra, onion, parsley, parsnip, pea, pumpkin, radish, rutabaga, salsify, spinach, sprouts (all kinds), squash (all kinds), Swiss chard, tomato, and turnip. You may also use the leaves or tops of beets, turnips, and the like. If you're not accustomed to raw food, too many different vegetables at a meal can be difficult to digest, so use fewer than four if necessary. If you wish, use a dressing of cold-pressed extra-virgin olive oil and lemon juice.
- **No coffee, tea, milk, or other beverages are permitted.**
- **No dessert.**

Before Dinner
- **Vegetable broth.** A half-hour before dinner, drink 2 cups of hot or cold vegetable broth This can be prepared in advance, as follows: finely chop beet, carrot, celery, green pepper, onion, parsley, zucchini, and thick peelings of potato (from the skin inward a half-inch, which is the part that's high in potassium); simmer for a half-hour in distilled water; strain to remove the solids, keeping the broth. If you wish, add fresh garlic to taste after straining.

Dinner
- **Fresh, raw vegetables.** Eat a chopped salad of up to four vegetables from the lunch list. If you wish, use a dressing of cold-pressed extra-virgin olive oil and lemon juice.
- **Steamed vegetables.** Also eat two or three vegetables steamed until tender but still crisp (about five minutes). If you wish, sprinkle with oregano, basil, dill, rosemary, thyme, or other unprocessed seasonings.
- **Bread.** Also eat one medium slice of whole-wheat bread (well toasted) or unleavened bread, plain.
- **No coffee, tea, milk, or other beverages are permitted.**
- **No dessert.**

After Dinner

- **Psyllium drink.** Two hours after dinner, drink 1 heaping teaspoon of psyllium seed powder mixed in 8 ounces of orange, pineapple, or apple juice.

Chapter 3
Creating Foundational Formulas for Healing

This book is not based on any single healing philosophy; instead, it synthesizes the healing arts. All therapies are good in some way at some times. My goal is to help you understand how your body speaks to you, and to educate you in modes of healing, so you can make better choices when you're not feeling well. Nothing takes the place of a good doctor, but a little education can go a long way, even if you only use it to choose the type of healer with whom you want to work.

The big question: what therapy to use and when? Turning to the same healer every time isn't best—you have to figure out what type(s) of physician to see for your particular problem. Sometimes a combination of therapies is useful. In most cases, you can do a lot for yourself while working with your doctor—so don't be afraid to explain that you're using nutrition or other modalities to enhance his/her suggested therapy. We've been conditioned to leave our health in the hands of a physician, but our health is our responsibility. You know your body better than anybody. Let knowledge be your guide.

This chapter discusses how the whole body is energetically and physiologically connected and how to determine what organs or systems need attention. It then explains how to use foods, herbs, and supplements to affect selected body functions and address your specific health issues, in an approach aligned with both Eastern and Western healing philosophies. And you don't have to study herbology, nutrition, Chinese medicine, biochemistry, or pathology—this book's charts and lists give you a head start on your health journey.

Meet Your Meridians

Chinese medicine has been telling us for 5,000 years that the whole body is connected through a system of energy pathways called meridians. The meridians travel on or near the skin and meet inside the body. The energy that flows through them influences all organs, systems, and bodily functions, and they can be used to diagnose and treat ailments.

Meridians can be blocked by infection, sickness, stress, scar tissue, tumors, congestion, and toxins. The current traveling through a blockage is weakened, and that affects the energy in the surrounding area. When energy isn't flowing properly, a problem in one organ can end up affecting another. A physician of traditional Chinese medicine can treat almost any disease by breaking up these blockages, restoring the body's energy circulation, and bringing the current back into balance. When acupuncturists needle certain patterns of points on the skin, they're using the meridians to affect and balance countless activities, from nervous system transmission and hormone secretion to nutrient transport and more.

Proof positive. The meridians' existence and location have been confirmed by modern scientific methods. In 1960, Professor Kim Bong Han injected radioactive phosphorous into a rabbit at specific acupuncture points and discovered that the isotope was actively taken up along the path of the classical acupuncture meridians. Researchers subsequently mapped the meridians and acupuncture points by taking readings from a wheel-shaped electrode rolled over the body's surface. These readings showed that acupuncture points act like little generators, sending out electrical currents that are conducted along the meridians and flow into the central nervous system.

The Academy of Clinical Acupuncture uses an instrument called a Ryodoraku to measure meridian energy levels by taking readings of human electromagnetic fields. By touching the probe to acupuncture points all over the body and graphing the readings, a practitioner can determine the exact location of energy imbalances. A high reading can indicate inflammation; a low reading, degeneration or blockage. *(Gerber R. Vibrational Medicine. Bear and Company, Santa Fe, NM, 1988; Becker R. The Body Electric. William Morrow, NY, 1985)*

Energy schedule. It's also been shown that energy flows predictably from one organ system to another in a specific circadian rhythm. Energy is always traveling throughout the body, and all organs always have energy—but at particular times in each 24-hour period, certain organs have more energy than at other times. These peak times are depicted below

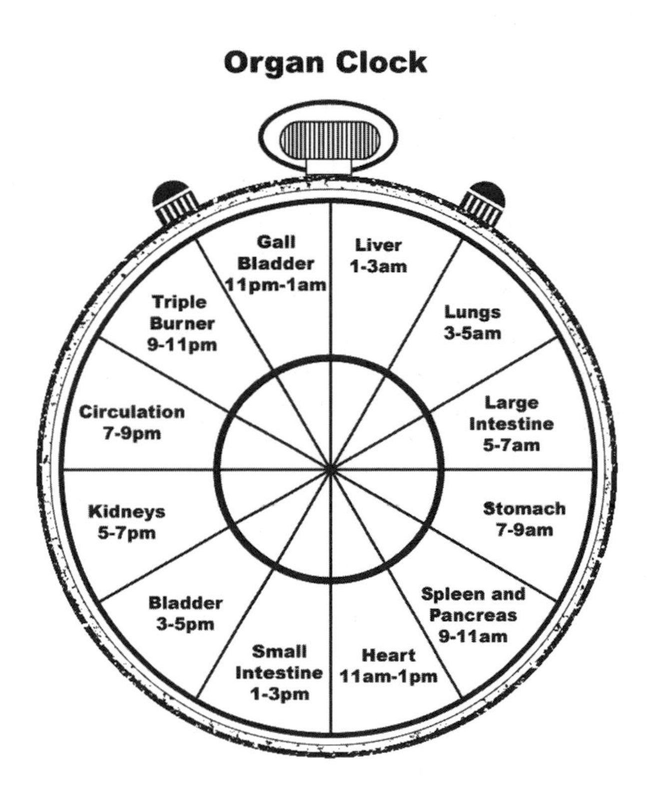

Referring to the Organ Clock may help locate the source of a health problem, because symptoms are often experienced during the affected organ's peak energy time. Let's say that around 1:00–3:00 a.m., you don't sleep well, perhaps with some digestive symptoms; according to the clock, that timing could indicate a liver issue, maybe with gallbladder involvement. In traditional Chinese medicine, the period of an organ's peak energy is also considered the best time to strengthen it, so treatment is often timed accordingly. An herbal compound for the lungs would be given between 3:00 and 5:00 a.m.; heart medicine, between 11:00 a.m. and 1:00 p.m.; a kidney remedy, 6:00–7:00 p.m. (Of course, working or sleeping may make it difficult or impossible to take a remedy at a certain time.)

Meridians and Symptoms

Your body can manifest physical symptoms if you are energetically "sick" due to a blocked meridian. A blockage in an energy pathway interferes with the proper flow of energy, nerve transmission, and nutrients along that pathway, and can also affect those connected to it. The resulting symptoms, however, may not be overtly recognizable or conventionally diagnosable. You could feel unwell, or have pain or a disturbed bodily function, but if the symptoms are subclinical, they may not be seen as anything more than the "I don't know why you're sick" syndrome—unless meridians are taken into account.

As an example, consider the liver meridian, which runs from the big toe up to the eyes. Let's say that the normal upward flow of energy in this meridian is blocked by calcium deposits built up around your long-ago ankle fracture, or by accumulated toxins in the liver—but you don't know about this blockage. What you do know is that you have knee pain, and yet as far as your doctor can tell, your knee is fine.

Maps and manifestations. Check out the following pictures to get an idea of the meridians' relationships, peak energy times, and associated symptoms (no need to memorize anything). You'll find it interesting, and maybe surprising—and a reminder of why we should always use a holistic approach to healing.

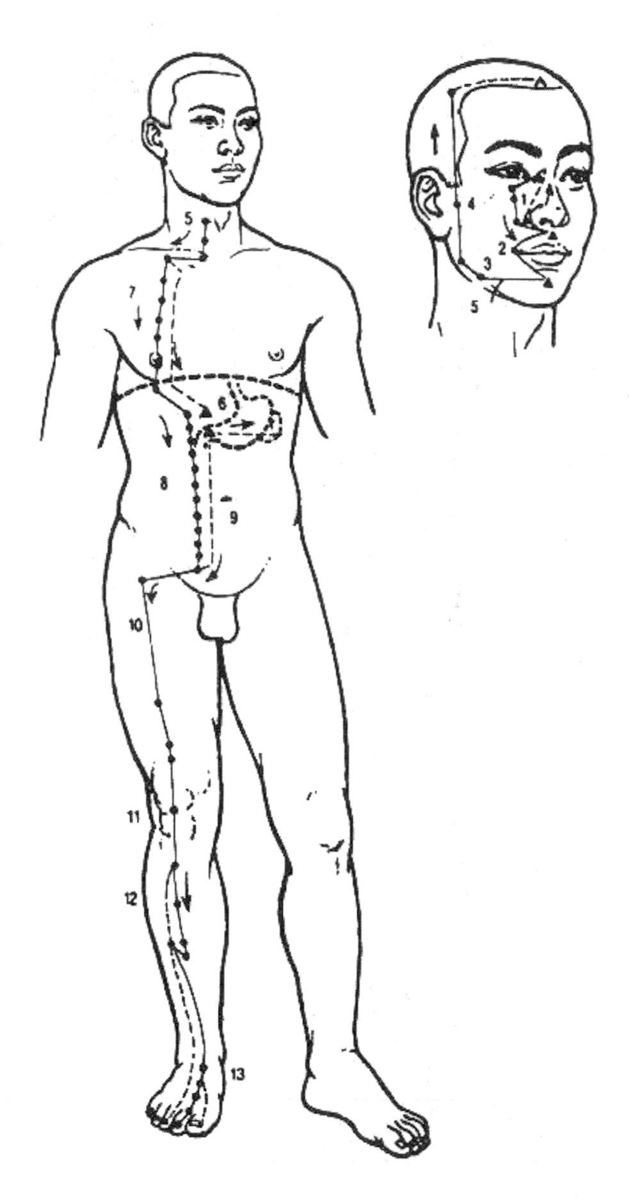

Stomach Meridian 7:00–9:00 a.m. Headache, sinus or throat or digestive problems, gastritis, hiatal hernia, ulcers, insufficient hydrochloric acid, bloating, pelvic or thigh or knee pain.

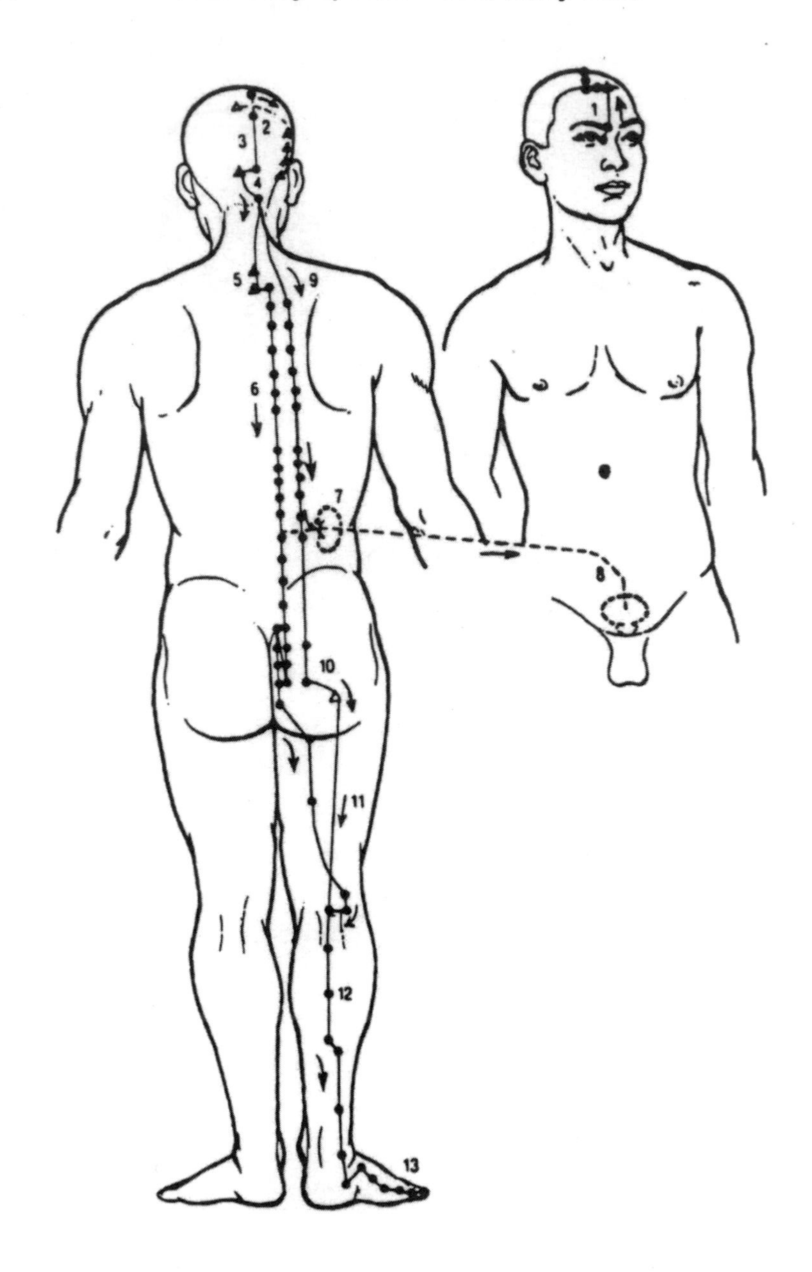

Bladder Meridian 3:00–5:00 p.m. Kidney or bladder infection, incontinence, painful or excessive urination, prostate or ovarian or uterine problems, sweating, hip or knee pain, leg or foot problems. Longest meridian.

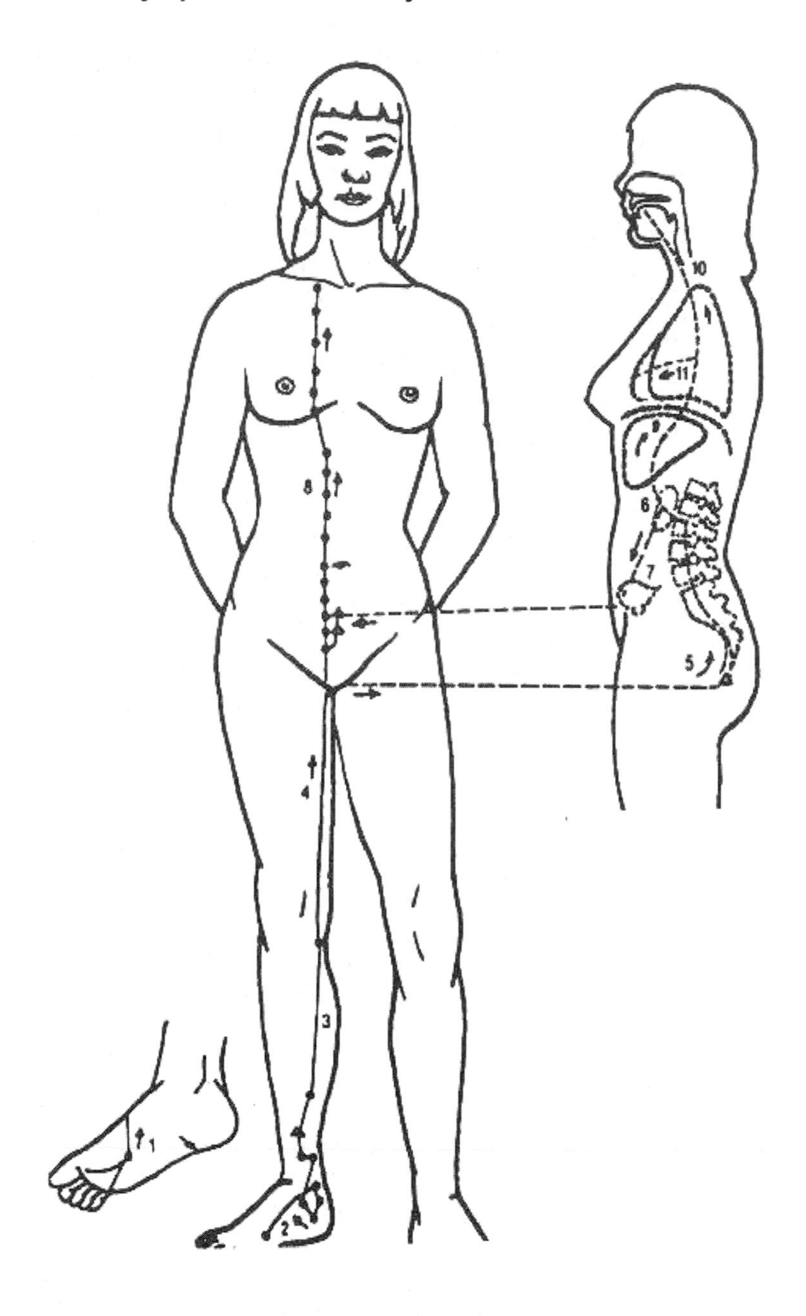

<u>Kidney Meridian</u> 5:00–7:00 p.m. Chronic ear problems, acute tinnitus, poor memory, dry mouth, dehydration, lung congestion, disc problems, lower back or hip or tailbone pain, hemorrhoids, knee or ankle pain. Controls hair growth on head.

MORE MERIDIANS AND ASSOCIATED SYMPTOMS

Liver Meridian 1:00–3:00 a.m. Eye problems, tendon or connective tissue problems, muscle or joint stiffness, eczema, psoriasis or dermatitis, arthritis, back pain, digestive problems.
Lung Meridian 3:00–5:00 a.m. Throat or vocal cord problems, shoulder or elbow pain, coughing, shortness of breath, chest or diaphragm tightness, bronchitis, asthma, emphysema, sweating, diarrhea, constipation, colitis.
Large Intestine Meridian 5:00–7:00 a.m. Sinus or nose or tooth problems, stiff neck or fingers, tennis elbow, abdominal bloating or pain, constipation, irritable bowel.
Spleen and Pancreas Meridian 9:00–11:00 a.m. Infection, immune system deficiency, lymphatic congestion, pancreas disturbance, diabetes, hypoglycemia. Sugar imbalances affect energies of all tissues. Spleen and pancreas also affect thyroid and adrenal glands, prostate, and ovaries (hormonal balance).
Heart Meridian 11:00 a.m.–1:00 p.m. Excessive emotions, dry hair or mouth, facial pain, nausea, palpitations, heart or blood vessel issues, chest or arm or mid-back pain, carpal tunnel syndrome, elbow or wrist pain, numbness, poor circulation, varicose veins, swollen ankles.
Small Intestine Meridian 1:00–3:00 p.m. Tinnitus, ear or throat problems, lateral shoulder or abdominal pain, diarrhea, intestinal flu, Crohn's disease.
Circulation/Sex Meridian 7:00–9:00 p.m. Depression, poor memory or concentration, sleep disorder, hormonal imbalance, chest or armpit pain, all heart problems, poor circulation, arteriosclerosis, hot flashes, sweaty palms, trembling. Governs relationship between pituitary gland and hypothalamus.
Triple Burner Meridian 9:00–11:00 p.m. Regulates temperature by controlling blood flow and water flow in three bodily divisions: upper (heart, lungs), middle (stomach, spleen, liver, gallbladder), and lower (kidneys, bladder, intestines). Tied to thyroid and adrenal gland function. Affects metabolism and digestive energy. Chronic fatigue, low energy, thinning hair, cataracts, ear infection, lasting colds, tonsillitis, body temperature too hot or too cold, cold hands or feet, hot flashes, menstrual irregularity.
Gallbladder Meridian 11:00 p.m.–1:00 a.m. Headache, nausea, tightness under right ribcage, muscle pain, digestive problems, bloating, gall stones.

Nutrition, Energy, and Coupled Organs

All foods, juices, herbs, and supplements function on two levels: the energetic and the physical. When the body absorbs nutrients and other substances, they influence the body's energy as well as the body's physiology. With the understanding that all organs and functions are interrelated—not only by nerves, hormones, and blood circulation, but also by meridians—you can see that a good nutritional program should support all bodily systems at both of those levels.

Nutrients are "departmentalized," meaning that each affects specific tissues, organs, and functions. Similarly, the energies of foods and herbs affect specific meridians. Why? Nature's design. All sciences, including nutrition, are based on fundamental natural laws. Electricity, for example, acts in a certain way, and nothing will change that. To perform the precise functions they were designed for, your organs need the energy and nutrients appropriate to them, and nothing will change that either.

Coupled therapy. As noted, the meridians are connected and link all organs energetically. Coupled organs (see below) are on similar energy pathways. Energy from one coupled organ flows toward the other, and they always work together.

COUPLED ORGANS

Kidneys/Bladder

Liver/Gallbladder

Lungs/Large Intestine

Stomach/Spleen/Pancreas

Heart/Small Intestine/Glands

Imbalance or dysfunction in an organ affects its coupled organ(s). In nutrition and herbology, as in acupuncture, when you treat an organ, you work with its coupled organ(s) at the same time. If you're working with the kidneys, you work with the bladder too. If you're working with the stomach, you also work with the spleen, and perhaps the pancreas—and so forth.

Likewise, when an organ shows symptoms, the whole body should be supported while specific therapies are undertaken for that priority organ and its coupled organ(s). For example, if your problem is constipation, the bowel is the priority organ, and it's coupled with the lungs, but aren't the other digestive organs involved, and influencing all of your systems? Of course.

Consider the case of nutritional therapy for a gallbladder problem. The gallbladder meridian travels from the eye to the big toe, so symptoms can arise at any place along that meridian—an eyesight issue, digestive trouble, knee pain. Its connected meridian, the liver meridian, can also be affected, and because the liver purifies the bloodstream, the original problem is thus connected to the entire body. I'd use nutritional treatments specific to the gallbladder and liver, and perhaps a cleanse for those two organs; meanwhile, I'd also provide foundational nutrition for the entire body, as described below. Targeting the priority and coupled organs while supporting the whole should help with the root problem—and who knows what other symptoms may clear up!

Foundational Nutrition

In supporting the entire body with nutrition that's foundational for good health, I usually suggest that people stay on two important supplements that work together: digestive enzymes and probiotics. No matter how clean your diet or lifestyle is, these are probably necessary. A failure in any health program can most likely be traced to a deficiency of enzymes and probiotics. Another important component of foundational nutrition is a whole-food or herbal supplement.

Enzymes. Supplemental enzymes provide very important support for the digestive system in general, and for the intestines and pancreas in particular. After the age of 30, most of us are deficient in one or more of the main digestive enzyme categories: protease for proteins, lipase for fats, amylase for carbohydrates and sugars, and cellulase to release the nutrients in fibers. Enzymes are produced in your body and occur naturally in raw foods, but if you eat cooked food or have a long-term history of eating cooked food, supplemental enzymes are necessary. Take them before meals in the quantity suggested on the package (if you eat meat, you may wish to take extra).

It's almost impossible to maintain normal vitamin and mineral balances without good digestion. Efficient digestion of protein and fat, for example, is critical for proper hormone levels and nerve function. I can't imagine trying to overcome any deficiencies or other health conditions without a normal digestive enzyme level to break down and release the building blocks from foods. My book *Food Enzymes: The Missing Link to Radiant Health (Hohm Press, Prescott, AZ, 1993)* explains how crucial enzymes are for weight loss, hormonal balance, athletics, and the control of allergies, hypoglycemia, and diabetes.

Probiotics. Probiotics—the name means "for life"—are bacteria such as lactobacillus that help maintain an important balance between beneficial and harmful microorganisms in the intestinal tract. You have 3–4 pounds of "friendly" and "unfriendly" microorganisms in there, and experts say you need 85 percent to be friendly to keep the remaining 15 percent at bay. The helpful bacteria assist with digestion, bowel pH and activity, and liver detoxification. They also stimulate the immune system, produce vitamin K and some B-vitamins, help prevent skin problems, and reduce cholesterol buildup.

Your internal bacterial balance can be upset by poor diet, coffee, antibiotics, drugs, stress, and other external influences. Bacterial imbalance in the bowel opens the door for infections and can produce a host of symptoms: acne, allergy, anxiety, bad breath, bloating, B-vitamin deficiency, and other fungal infection, cold or flu, constipation, depression, diarrhea, fatigue, fibromyalgia, flatulence, high cholesterol, itchy skin, muscle pain, premenstrual syndrome, psoriasis, tension headache, and urinary tract infection.

Take your probiotic supplement on an empty stomach. Some foods containing friendly bacteria are fermented milk products, cultured dairy products such as yogurt and kefir, fermented pickles, and sauerkraut. To stimulate probiotic growth, eat "prebiotic" carbohydrates called oligosaccharides—soluble, nondigestible fibers naturally found in whole grains, fruits, vegetables, and legumes. Particularly prebiotic-rich foods are chicory, dandelion green, flaxseed, garlic, leek, and onion.

Juice Plus+®. A whole-food supplement that supports all of the meridians, Juice Plus+® is the most studied nutraceutical in the world today. Its ingredients, demonstrated benefits, and role in foundational nutrition are detailed in chapters 4 and 5. But whatever whole-food or herbal supplement you choose, be sure there's primary research behind it, as there is for Juice Plus+®—that's research on the effects of its ingredients in combination, not separately. Not all foods or herbs work well together.

More digestion tips. A problem in any digestive organ affects your digestion of food and absorption of nutrients. To address difficulties in these areas, always consider taking supplemental enzymes and probiotics, then add more green foods to your diet, or try green powders such as wheatgrass, chlorella, barley grass, spirulina, and kamut.

For general digestive support and for constipation, plenty of fiber and water are important. For diarrhea, the green foods and powders are helpful, as are pectin-rich foods such as apple, blueberry, carrot, and grapefruit—carob powder is especially good in children. Enzymes and probiotics are helpful against both diarrhea and constipation. For circulatory issues related to digestion, onion and garlic have demonstrated benefits in lowering blood sugar, cholesterol, and pressure.

Additional dietary guidelines are given later in this chapter.

The Balancing and Healing Chart

The Balancing and Healing Chart below illustrates your body's physiological and energetic interconnections. The circles contain coupled organs and related tissues, and the arrows represent the energy cycles in Chinese medicine. For the non-physician and non-acupuncturist, it's an easy way to see how the body works.

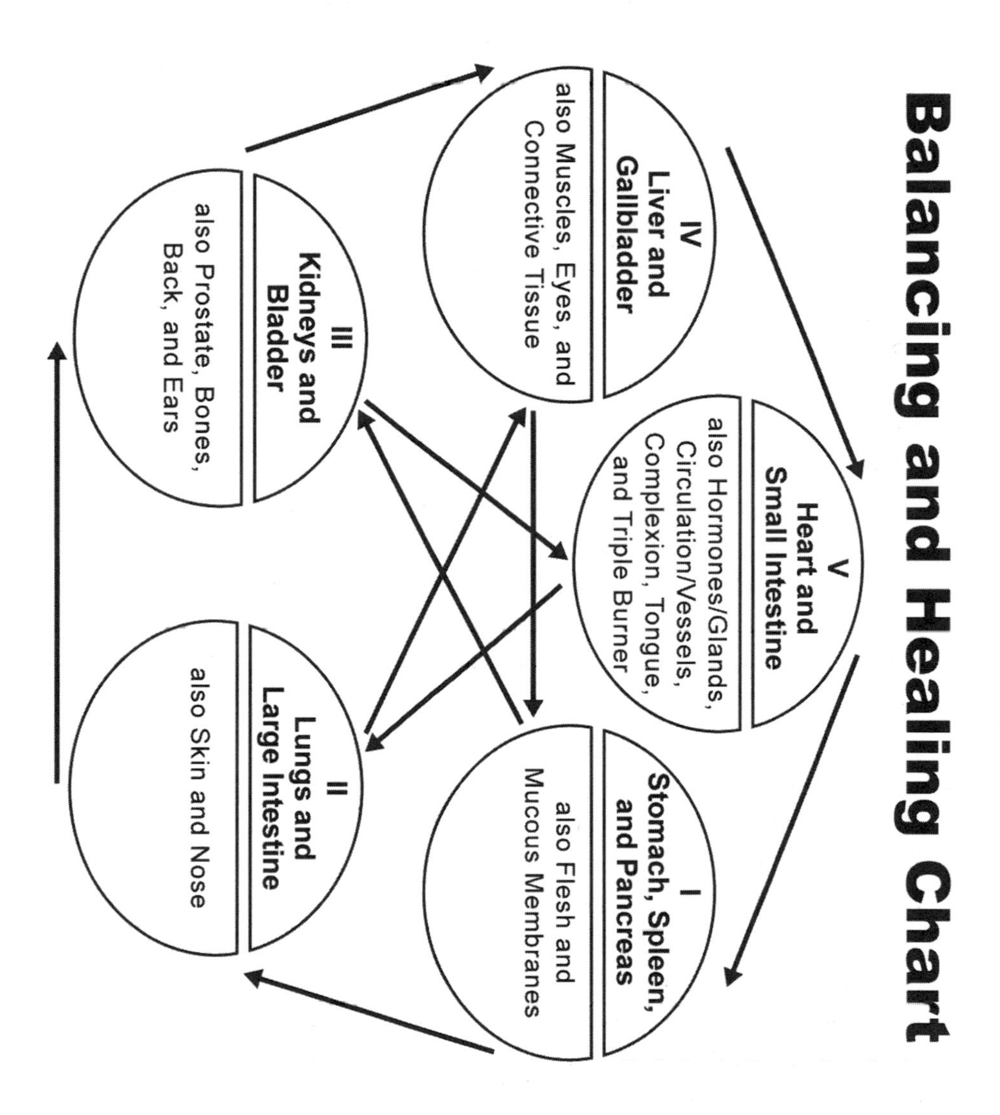
Balancing and Healing Chart
I
Stomach, Spleen, and Pancreas
also Flesh and Mucous Membranes
II
Lungs and Large Intestine
also Skin and Nose
III
Kidneys and Bladder
also Prostate, Bones, Back, and Ears
IV
Liver and Gallbladder
also Muscles, Eyes, and Connective Tissue
V
Heart and Small Intestine
also Hormones/Glands, Circulation/Vessels, Complexion, Tongue, and Triple Burner

Going with the flow. The outer arrows, called the Generation Cycle, represent the flow of energy from each set of organs and tissues to the next, sometimes called the "mother-son" relationship. Circle I "feeds" energy to circle II, which feeds circle III, and so on. But with dysfunction or disease, the energy does not flow properly. If energy is blocked by something, the organ or area "downstream" suffers from decreased energy or blood flow. If an organ is weak or imbalanced, it draws too much energy from the organs before it and may not send enough on to the next. For example, a weak liver can drain the kidneys and be unable to feed the heart. Excess energy held up in an organ or area can cause inflammation and pain, possibly becoming a chronic disease as time goes on.

The inner arrows are the Control Cycle, representing bloodstream and nervous system connections as well as energy flow. These arrows indicate that each organ has some control over another, for better or for worse. For example, the inner arrow from the kidneys to the heart means that weak kidneys weaken the heart, as when fluid retention leads to a heart problem, and strong kidneys strengthen the heart. Now look at both arrows coming from the heart, and you can see that a strong heart strengthens the lungs (inner arrow) as well as the stomach, spleen, and pancreas (outer arrow). In this way, all organs support each other—or, can weaken each other.

If you take a medication for a particular health problem, you can check the Balancing and Healing Chart to shed light on possible side effects. For example, you may have heard of kidney medication affecting eyesight, strangely enough; that's because of the mother-son relationship of circle III, containing the kidneys, to circle IV, containing the eyes. You can minimize a medication's side effects by supporting the potentially affected organs with appropriate nutrition and herbs.

A New Way of Healing: The Triad Approach

Western medical specialists tend to divide the body into parts for diagnosis and treatment, but Eastern philosophies of medicine pay attention to the whole. No matter what the health problem is, there's a way to strengthen the whole body while working on that specific problem. When all bodily connections are supported while a dominant symptom is addressed, healing happens in a shorter time—and that's when we see miracles. This is how chronic conditions must be treated.

I've developed an approach to healing based on that principle, utilizing the Balancing and Healing Chart. I call it Triad Healing, because for any specific imbalance or health problem, a triad from the chart—three circles, linked by the inner arrows—is used to create targeted therapeutic formulas of foods and herbs. Ultimately, treating a triad also supports the other two circles, as they're all linked by the outer arrows.

This healing approach has three steps:

1. Identify Your Triad of Interest

To identify your triad, you start by identifying your priority organ, according to the specific health issue you want to work on, and find that priority organ in the chart. Then you follow the inner arrow from that circle to the next circle, and again to the next circle, and those three circles are your triad of interest.

To illustrate, let's say the health issue is asthma, so you start at your priority organ, the lungs, in circle II. Follow the inner arrow from circle II to circle IV, and the next inner arrow to circle I, and that's the triad for this example: lungs/large intestine, liver/gallbladder, and stomach/spleen/pancreas.

2. Create a Food Formula

Now build a therapeutic formula for your triad from the list of Foods for Organ Support at the end of this chapter. Starting with your priority organ, select two items from the food group for that organ. Then select one or two for the second circle in your triad, and another one or two for the third circle. Each of these foods does not need to be different—in fact, it's helpful to use foods that support more than one organ in your triad.

Continuing the asthma example to illustrate, I'll start with the food group for the lungs, and choose garlic and spinach. Those also happen to be listed for the coupled organ, the large intestine. For the next triad circle, liver/gallbladder, I'll choose parsley from the liver group. I see that my first selection, spinach, is in the liver group too, so I'll move on to the third triad circle. I see that the spinach and parsley I already chose are listed for stomach/spleen/pancreas too, so I don't have to make another selection, but I want to, so I choose beet and apple from the stomach and spleen groups. Beet is also listed for the gallbladder and lungs; overlap is good. My formula is:

- Lungs/large intestine—garlic, spinach
- Liver/gallbladder—parsley
- Stomach/spleen/pancreas—beet, apple

Your selected foods can be juiced, blended, or eaten in a salad or other concoction. Whatever form you choose for your formula, it should always include two or more foods that affect your priority organ. And as noted above, it's good to include foods that are common to more than one of the organs you're working with. It's easy to have variety by changing your selections from one formula to the next—and this is a good idea, as the types, amounts, and combinations of thousands of beneficial nutrients vary from food to food.

Take your food formula two or three times a day as a part of your diet, not as a replacement for it. As a general guideline, continue taking it for 7–14 days after your health condition has cleared. If you juice or blend your formula, I suggest a dose of 8–12 ounces at a time; and if you're doing a lot of juicing, I recommend using no more than four foods per combination. When I juice or blend, I always add an apple for taste. Ginger is good for taste too, plus it acts as a carrier for other nutrients.

3. Create an Herbal Formula

In choosing herbs for additional support, you have a few options. You can get a prepared herbal combination for your specific health issue from a health food store or an herbalist; you can use my book *Natural Healing with Herbs (Hohm Press, Prescott, AZ, 1984),* which describes formulas for 133 conditions; or you can build an herbal formula for your triad from the list of Herbs for Organ and System Support at the end of this chapter.

As with the foods, you'll notice that many herbs have an effect on more than one organ. Continuing with the asthma example to illustrate, your formula could be:

- Lungs/large intestine—fenugreek, mullein
- Liver/gallbladder—milk thistle
- Stomach/spleen/pancreas—goldenseal

Herbs are typically taken as capsules, tinctures, and infusions (strong tea). If you build a formula yourself, you probably won't actually combine your herbs into a single mixture as you do with your foods; they may be in different forms, and their recommended number of doses per day may differ. In any case, always use more herbs directed toward your priority organ than toward your other two triad circles. After your condition clears, continue taking your herbs for another week or as advised by an experienced practitioner.

I suggest adding ginger to any infusion, for taste and as a carrier for the active substances in the herbs. For additional cleansing when working with any triad, I suggest 3 cups daily of dandelion tea—dandelion's listed for several organs.

Sometimes it's easier to buy a combination herbal product. If you do that, it's important to check the product against the herb list to make sure that the product covers the triad you want to support. Get professional guidance if necessary.

See? It's easy, fun, and healing. This approach can also be utilized alongside other therapies suggested by your health practitioner or of your own choosing, such as homeopathy. Triad Healing is a way to really help yourself, especially if you do a little reading about foods and herbs. That's what it's all about—taking control of your health, happiness, and future.

Two More Triad Formulating Examples

A kidney problem. First the triad: starting at the kidneys, circle III, across to circulation/small intestine, circle V, and across again to lungs/large intestine, circle II. Then go to the food list: for the priority organ, the kidneys (coupled with the bladder), you could choose dandelion and parsley; for circulation/small intestine, beet and cucumber; and for lungs/large intestine, carrot and romaine. Then go to the herb list: for kidneys/bladder, you could choose burdock and cleavers; for circulation/small intestine, yarrow; and for lungs/large intestine, flaxseed. If you are also constipated, use *Cascara sagrada* for three to five days or consult a physician.

A liver problem. Triad: start at the liver in circle IV, go across to circle I, and across again to circle III. Possible food formula: for liver/gallbladder, carrot and watercress; for stomach/spleen/pancreas, parsley; and for kidneys/bladder, endive. Possible herbal formula: for liver/gallbladder, milk thistle and red clover; for stomach/spleen/pancreas, goldenseal; and for kidneys/bladder, dandelion.

Breaking the Toxic Cycle in Your Primary Triad

The "primary triad" is the large intestine, liver/gallbladder, and stomach/spleen—and it's often a toxic triad. A domino effect occurs when the overload of toxins in any of these organs is passed on to the next and the next and eventually dumped into the bloodstream, affecting the whole body. This toxic cycle is another example of how all body parts and functions are related—and how degeneration and chronic disease develop.

Some experts say 90 percent of all disease starts in the colon. The colon is the main channel of elimination of harmful bacteria, parasites, waste, medication, and other toxins. But over time, hardened fecal matter builds up on the colon wall, impeding the absorption of nutrients and the exit of bad microbes and waste. Normal daily bowel movements don't necessarily mean the colon is clean—and if it isn't, toxic substances can be reabsorbed into the body. (Plus, isn't it absurd to spend money on supplements if your colon can't take them in?)

When inadequate digestion overtaxes the liver and bowel, the toxin overload is sent through the kidneys. Toxins that the overstressed kidneys can't handle go back into the bloodstream and are carried to the lungs. Toxins that the lungs can't expel through exhalation re-enter the bloodstream and are dumped into the lymphatic system, causing toxic lymph fluid, swollen lymph nodes, and stress on the spleen. Acids build up in the blood, taxing the immune system and encouraging infections. These accumulated poisons disturb the pH of the fluids surrounding the cells, so the connective tissue becomes toxic, possibly leading to inflammatory syndromes such as fibromyalgia and arthritis. The poisons in the lymph and blood can also affect and even damage the heart. At this point, you may need to see a doctor!

The only way to get out of this mess before it goes too far is to back up and address the history of these conditions by detoxifying the body and correcting the functions of the primary triad. It takes time, money, and patience to break that toxic cycle, but you can do it. My suggestions are below. *Note:* Don't do what I first did, which was all of the following at once—I had ten bowel movements a day and spent hours in the bathroom.

Diet and digestion are foremost. There are plenty of books on dietary improvement, and you'll find a full treatment of the subject in *ProMetabolics*. For the purposes of this book, and life in general, my primary dietary suggestions are:

- Cut out sugar, heavy dairy products, and high-carb foods.
- You certainly know what junk food is, so cut that out too.
- Eat fruits, vegetables, sprouted grains, and lean meats (unless you're a vegetarian).

- Study proper food combinations.
- Keep your meals simple.
- Drink plenty of pure water.
- Don't eat after 7:00 p.m.

You can start cleansing your toxic triad by using the purification diet in chapter 2. If you have a problem with sugar, limit the fruits. Add lean meats and fish if you'd like.

A very important part of this first step is to support your digestion and improve any eliminative symptoms by taking supplemental enzymes and probiotics as described previously, so waste and fermenting food won't accumulate in your intestine. Take enzymes before every meal, and take probiotics on an empty stomach first thing in the morning and before bed.

Bowel cleanse. Next, you need a good bowel cleaning. I've done this for more than 20 years with the help of Sonne's No. 7 (available at health food stores or www.sonnes.com), a bentonite clay that absorbs 100 times its weight in toxins and accumulated intestinal mucus. For 14 consecutive days, take a good fiber such as psyllium seed with Sonne's No. 7 on an empty stomach in the morning and evening (follow the dose on the label). Wait a month, and then do it again. If the bowel doesn't move twice daily during this cleanse, take an herbal laxative in the evening, especially for bloating and gas. Colonics are also suggested.

Cleansing food formula. From the list of Foods for Organ Support, create a cleansing formula for the primary triad. If you're working with a health practitioner or experienced in detoxifying, you can use the food formula during the bowel cleanse period; otherwise, use it afterward. Here's an example of a cleansing formula for this triad:

- Large intestine— mustard green, spinach, watercress
- Liver/gallbladder—carrot, dandelion green, parsley
- Stomach/spleen—cabbage

Taken as juice or salad, these greens are all good blood purifiers and lymphatic cleansers; they also support the kidneys and their pH-balancing activities. Combined with the digestive enzymes assisting the stomach, spleen, and pancreas, now you have a thorough digestion-improvement program.

Liver/gallbladder cleanse. Fats and accumulated waste cause liver congestion and gallstones. Once you've done a bowel cleanse, you've cleared the way for a liver/gallbladder cleanse, long recommended by nutritionists and naturopaths as an annual practice for people over the age of 25. Before you start, make sure your energy level is increasing and you're strong enough to handle another cleanse. The method below has several components, followed for a three- to six-day period:

- Take a good herbal combination for the liver and gallbladder, such as Pure Encapsulation's LVR Formula (available through Mountain States Health Products, www.mhpvitamins.com), to support liver function and promote bile flow.
- Take 10 drops of Ultra P.P.I. (also available through MHP) in water three times daily or as directed by your physician. Ultra P.P.I. is orthophosphoric acid and inositol, which help soften and dissolve gallstones and cholesterol.
- Drink organic apple juice daily between meals, for a total of 2 quarts across the day.
- Take Juice Plus+ Garden Blend® and/or Vineyard Blend®, described in chapters 4 and 5.
- Eat a cleansing diet. Avoid bread, pasta, and other high-carb foods. If you use the purification diet in chapter 2, eliminate the bread at dinner.
- Drink plenty of water, at least six glasses daily.
- When you get up in the morning, take 2–3 teaspoons of magnesium citrate or disodium phosphate; if you don't have a bowel movement in a few hours, repeat this. Watch your stools for greenish globules or stones that may pass.
- Take 2–3 teaspoons of magnesium citrate or disodium phosphate between breakfast and lunch or between lunch and dinner, to keep your bowels moving. If you get diarrhea, back off to a lesser amount that will still assure two bowel movements daily.

- When you go to bed, lie on your right side with your knees pulled up to your chest for 30 minutes before sleeping.
- At bedtime on the final day, drink 4 ounces of cold-pressed virgin olive oil on an empty stomach. Follow this with some fresh grapefruit juice or cranberry juice to prevent nausea; if any, it'll disappear in less than an hour.

Kidney follow-up. After the liver/gallbladder cleanse, continue on your herbal formula and add a kidney cleanser for two months. I use MHP's Kidney Liquid, a homeopathic drainage remedy that works fantastically well. And there you have it! The cleansing of your primary triad is accomplished.

FOODS FOR ORGAN SUPPORT

Heart
Cilantro
Dandelion green
Green bean
Green grape
Lime

Circulation (Heart)
Acorn squash
Beet
Cucumber
Ginger
Radish
Red cabbage
Red pepper
Romaine
Strawberry

Bladder
Blueberry
Broccoli
Celery
Greens
Lemon
Lettuce
Mustard green
Onion
Orange
Parsley
Red grape
Romaine
Spinach
Turnip

Gallbladder

Gallbladder
Beet
Beet green
Bok choy
Dandelion green
Endive
Green bean
Kale
Mustard green
Plum
Radish
Strawberry
Sweet potato
Watercress

Kidneys

Kidneys
Beet
Dandelion green
Endive
Ginger
Grapefruit
Green pepper
Parsley
Watermelon
Zucchini

Large Intestine

Large Intestine
Bok choy
Butternut squash
Cherry
Garlic
Mustard green
Spinach
Tomato
Watercress

Liver

Liver
Carrot
Dandelion green
Endive
Grapefruit
Lettuce
Parsley
Spinach
Tomato
Watercress

Lungs

Lungs
Carrot
Cilantro
Garlic
Ginger
Green grape
Lime
Pineapple
Radish
Red potato
Romaine
Spinach
Strawberry
White potato

Pancreas

Acorn squash
Celery
Cucumber
Garlic
Green bean
Onion
Parsley
Radish
Romaine
Spinach
Sweet potato
Turnip
Watercress
Zucchini

Small Intestine

Green grape
Kale
Nectarine
Pear
Romaine
Spinach
Zucchini

Spleen

Apple
Beet
Beet green
Cranberry
Garlic
Lettuce
Parsley
Radish
Red cabbage
Red pepper
Tomato
Watercress

Stomach

Grapefruit
Green cabbage
Kiwi
Parsley
Pear
Radish
Red cabbage

Thyroid/Adrenals

Apple
Bok choy
Garlic
Ginger
Kale
Parsley
Strawberry
Turnip

HERBS FOR ORGAN AND SYSTEM SUPPORT

ADRENAL GLANDS
LICORICE
- 1 cup tea 2x day or
- 1–2 capsules 3x day

BAD BREATH
CLOVE
- chew 3–6 cloves as needed

SPEARMINT, PEPPERMINT
- 1 cup tea 3x day

BLADDER
BUCHU, NETTLES, PARSLEY, CLEAVERS, CORN SILK
- 1 cup tea 3x day

BLOOD
ALFALFA, BURDOCK, CLEAVERS, DANDELION, RED CLOVER
- 1 cup tea 3x day or
- 2 capsules 3x day

BONES
COMFREY
- 1 cup tea 3x day or
- 2 capsules 3x day

CIRCULATION
CAYENNE, GINKGO BILOBA
- as directed on label or by practitioner

GINGER, GINSENG, SASSAFRAS, SPEARMINT, YARROW
- 1 cup tea 3x day or
- 2 capsules 3x day

CONSTIPATION
CASCARA SAGRADA
- 2 capsules before bed 2–3 nights in a row

FLAXSEED
- 2 Tbsp. powder per day

PSYLLIUM SEED
- 1 tsp. powder in 8 oz. juice 2–3x day

DIARRHEA

BARBERRY
- 2 capsules between meals 2x day

GOLDENSEAL
- 2 capsules between or with meals 2–3x day

DIGESTIVE SUPPORT

GENTIAN
- 2 capsules between meals 2–3x day

EYES (eye strain)

EYEBRIGHT, FENNEL, GOLDENSEAL
- 1 cup tea 3x day or
- 2 capsules 3x day

FEMALE REPRODUCTIVE SYSTEM

CRAMPBARK, DAMIANA
- 1 cup tea 3x day or
- 2 capsules 3x day

GALLBLADDER

DANDELION, PARSLEY
- 1 cup tea 3x day or
- 2 capsules 3x day

HEADACHE

WHITE WILLOW BARK
- 2 capsules as needed

HEART

HAWTHORNE BERRY
- 2 capsules 3x day

INTESTINES (see also Constipation, Diarrhea)

BARBERRY, GOLDENSEAL, OREGON GRAPE
- natural intestinal antibiotic, as directed by practitioner, must be professionally monitored

---

JOINTS

DEVIL'S CLAW, COMFREY
- 2 capsules 3x day

KIDNEYS

BURDOCK, CLEAVERS, DANDELION, JUNIPER BERRY, SHEPHERD'S PURSE

- 1 cup tea 3x day or
- 2 capsules 3x day

LIVER

BARBERRY

- 2 capsules before meals 2–3x day

DANDELION, GOLDENSEAL, MILK THISTLE, PARSLEY, RED CLOVER

- 1 cup tea 3x day or
- 2 capsules 3x day

LUNGS

FENUGREEK, GARLIC, LICORICE, MULLEIN

- 1 cup tea 3x day or
- 2 capsules 3x day

LYMPHATIC SYSTEM

ECHINACEA, RED CLOVER

- 25–60 drops tincture in 1 cup water 3x day or
- 1 cup tea 3x day or
- 2 capsules 3x day

MALE REPRODUCTIVE SYSTEM

FO-TI, RED AMERICAN GINSENG, SAW PALMETTO BERRY

- 2 capsules 3x day

MUCOUS MEMBRANES (sore throat; see also Sinuses)

GOLDENSEAL, SAGE

- 1 cup tea 3x day or
- 2 capsules 3x day

MUSCLE ACHE

COMFREY

- 1 cup tea 3x day or
- 2 capsules 3x day

NERVOUS SYSTEM

CHAMOMILE, LADY'S SLIPPER, PLEURISY ROOT, SKULLCAP
- 1 cup tea 3x day or
- 2 capsules 3x day

PANCREAS (blood sugar issues, diabetes, diabetic retinopathy)

Note: Herb use for diabetes should be professionally monitored.

BILBERRY EXTRACT, GRAPE SEED EXTRACT
- as directed by practitioner

DANDELION, GREEN TEA
- 1 cup tea 2–3x day

FENUGREEK SEED
- 50 g defatted powder between meals 2x day

GYMNEMA SYLVESTRE
- as directed on label or by practitioner (usually 400 mg per day)

PROSTATE

PARSLEY, SAW PALMETTO BERRY
- 1 cup tea 3x day or
- 2 capsules 3x day

SINUSES (congestion)

GARLIC, GOLDENSEAL, SAGE
- 1 cup tea 3x day or
- 2 capsules 3x day

HORSERADISH
- 1/2 tsp. freshly grated root as needed, mixed with greens or with apple cider vinegar and water and a pinch of cayenne, or simply held in the mouth for several minutes

---

SKIN

RED CLOVER
- 1 cup tea 3x day

SPLEEN

GENTIAN, GOLDENSEAL, YELLOW DOCK
- 2 capsules 3x day

STOMACH

ALFALFA, CHAMOMILE, DANDELION, FENNEL, GINGER
- 1 cup tea 3x day or
- 2 capsules 3x day

Chapter 4

Juice Plus+®: How It Enhances Health and Supports Healing

Juice Plus+® offers three main products: the original Garden Blend® and Orchard Blend®, and now the Vineyard Blend®. Collectively, they comprise 23 concentrated fruit and vegetable juice powders, along with selected enzymes, phytonutrients, acidophilus culture, vitamins, minerals, and bran from two grains. Juice Plus+® is the best-selling encapsulated product and the most researched nutraceutical in the world today.

Popular among doctors and laypersons alike, Juice Plus+® is foundational nutrition used by all types of health practitioners. It can serve as a baseline foundational supplement to support all therapies, as well as to improve the body's utilization of other supplements. This chapter brings energetics, medical pathology, Chinese medicine, and other natural healing disciplines together in a holistic picture of how and why Juice Plus+® works so well.

Energy and Nutrition

Remember your high school chemistry? Fundamentally, everything is energy. Atoms are tiny energy packages, in which negatively charged electrons spin 600 miles per second around a nucleus containing neutrons and positively charged protons. As electrons whirl in their orbits, they generate an electromagnetic field. That field determines how the atom will attract or repel other electron configurations and join with other atoms to form molecules. Similarly, molecules attract and repel other molecules. The universe is made up of atoms, which make up molecules, which make up everything. Everything in the universe, from the elements on up, has an energetic matrix that is unique to its substance, and everything acts in a certain way.

Eating energy. All biochemical reactions are governed by the laws of energy, and the energetics of food is the basis of nutritional science. Each food has a characteristic physical structure made up of various substances including identified and unidentified nutrients—there can be more than 10,000 phytochemicals (plant chemicals) in one fruit or vegetable—as well as a characteristic energetic matrix. Additionally, the food's color and physical structure combined produce a specific vibration, which is the movement of the smallest particles.

The body can utilize the unique energy and nutritional content of all foods. Specific nutrients, however, are attracted to specific tissues—blood, bones, nerves, you name it—and specific foods affect specific organs. For example, vitamin A always goes to the liver, and calcium to the bones. Cranberry affects the kidneys and bladder, beet affects the liver, and prune affects the bowel. (Toxins behave similarly; mercury, for instance, goes to fatty tissue, including the brain, which is 60 percent fat.)

Bioavailability. One of my medical textbooks states, "Living organisms take up and release matter and energy during metabolism. Use of food molecules for energy requires that their molecular bonds be broken down." Two aspects again, energy and matter—and the body uses both continuously. *(Groër MW, Shekleton ME. Basic Pathophysiology: A Conceptual Approach. CV Mosby Company, St. Louis, MO, 1983)*

Processing and cooking foods not only destroys nutrients but also changes the foods' physical matrix, their energetic structure, and the natural synergy of their components, often making it difficult for the body to use them. Nutrients have specific relationships with each other. That synergy has a lot to do with their bioavailability—how well they're absorbed—and their utilization in the body.

I'm not saying you have to eat only raw foods or become a vegetarian; those ways of eating are an individual decision. What I am saying is that we all need whole-food supplements to complement our diets and support our bodies with bioavailable nutrients. This is where Juice Plus+® comes in. The foods and other ingredients in Juice Plus+® weren't thrown randomly into a capsule; rather, the formulas were carefully designed and combined in very specific ratios that are ideal for absorption and use by the human body.

The Birth of Juice Plus+®

Before I tell you about the research behind Juice Plus+®, I'd like to tell you the personal story that led to the development of this whole-food product. When we're experiencing a trauma or other significant event, we don't always fully understand it until it has passed, and then we realize that it has changed our lives for the better. Living a life is a lesson itself and is always teaching us something; we just have to learn how to interpret the direction that it's taking us. Even a chronic illness is pointing us in a specific direction, as I learned when my father got sick.

It was 1980 and I was on a lecture tour, teaching herbal seminars in Denver, Colorado. During a break, I received a phone call from my father. He told me his spleen had swollen to the size of a football. It was so large he was using one of his Marine Corps belts to hold it up, and it was so painful that he could hardly move. My mother made an appointment for him at a nearby hospital, where the doctors could not believe how large his spleen had grown—and it was still growing.

At the end of the day, my dad called me again and said he was diagnosed with lymphoma, cancer of the lymphatic system. I was so stunned I couldn't even reply. I just held the phone, praying that I didn't really hear what he had said. My throat closed up, so tight I could hardly breathe. He felt my shock and distress and told me everything was going to be okay. Being a naturopath and teaching people for years how to live by the laws of nature, I had to ask myself, why did this have to happen? (Don't we all wonder why, when something so traumatic happens to us?)

I told my dad I'd be home in four days, as soon as my tour was over. By the time I got there, his doctors had already removed his spleen and started chemotherapy. I was floored, totally irate. No questions had been asked—they just did the surgery and started pumping him full of drugs.

After three weeks, my father had lost 40 pounds and nothing was working. The chemotherapy had failed, and there was nothing more they could do. His doctor called our family together and told us my dad had no more than three weeks to live. After breaking the news to my dad, I asked if he'd like to try natural therapy at my clinic in Tucson, where I would take care of him. He said, "I would have come to you before this, but I didn't want you to be responsible if anything bad would have happened to me." I picked him up and carried him out of the hospital without even checking him out.

By the time we got to Tucson, he weighed 136 pounds, and his cancer was traveling so fast through his body that he couldn't eat or drink. How do you nourish somebody who can't eat or drink? I started massaging him every day with olive oil so his body would absorb the fat through his skin. He could only sip water, so I devised a plan to get more nutrients in through another route. I built a slant board for him to lie on, made fresh green juice with kale, parsley, and some additional liquid chlorophyll, and used an enema bag to feed him through the bowel with this juice daily.

As he got stronger, he was able to drink vegetable juices by mouth. Fruit juices, however, made him feel ill because of their sugar. You don't want to feed cancer cells sugar, because they thrive on it; plus, it acidifies the body, putting an even greater strain on a sick person's system.

I wanted to find a way to get more concentrated nutrition into his body to increase his strength and boost his healing, and it occurred to me that if I could juice the vegetables and dry the juice, the powder would be more concentrated than the juice itself. I set up some small dryers in my office and found that it took hours to dry the juice, but it worked. I gave him tablespoons of vegetable juice powder stirred into small amounts of water daily. To my amazement—keep in mind, at that time we knew nothing about phytochemicals—in two months he put on 30 pounds. There was no meat and no carbohydrate other than tablespoons of dried vegetable juice in his diet. I wondered, how could someone put on so much weight without eating?

He then got to the point where he could also drink fruit juice powder without feeling ill, so he had fruit juice powder in the morning and vegetable juice powder the rest of the day. I gave him very little fruit juice powder, though, as I noticed that giving him too much made his urine's pH acidic. I also added proteolytic enzymes and some herbs to the regime. I was constantly changing the dosages of his supplements according to his pH, using the monitoring system described in my book *ProMetabolics.*

The results were astonishing. Within three months of my taking over his treatment, my father got out of bed and remodeled my kitchen. He had been a carpenter his whole life and loved working with wood. Continuing on a nutritional program of eating large amounts of vegetables, dried juice powders, and soaked and sprouted seeds and nuts, he went back to work within six months and worked as a carpenter for another six years. It's my opinion that he'd still be alive today if his doctors had not removed his spleen and given him such high doses of drugs during his hospitalization.

From my father's recovery, I realized the hidden healing power of whole foods, so I began studying all fruits and vegetables known to man, and I discovered that some were much more nutrient-dense than others. The ones most concentrated in nutrients were the ones most people didn't eat at all, or always cooked before eating: parsley, beets, cabbage, and broccoli, to name a few. Experimenting with several fruits and vegetables over several months, I designed one concentrated powder formula with fruits and another with vegetables. These two formulas contained an array of the most nutrient-dense fruits and vegetables on the planet.

By this time my clinic looked more like a drying facility for fruit and vegetable juice powders, and everyone who came to me, regardless of the problem, was given a bag of each powder. The healings that I observed were no less than miraculous. I knew I was on to something big when my patients were getting well so fast. I quickly contacted a patent attorney, but it took five years to get the patent on my idea, which I received on my birthday. That was significant to me because I believe that everything that happens to us is God-sent, a gift to receive and learn from.

The formulas that I used for those years in my clinical practice are now called Juice Plus+®. I designed and patented this product, and NSA, Inc. (Memphis, TN) manufactured, distributed, and promoted it. Today, these God-given products are benefiting thousands of people in more than thirty countries.

Just before my father died, he was so concerned about my professional reputation that he said, "If I die, will people still believe in you? Will they still buy your books?" I said, "Dad, what we accomplished together, this idea of concentrated fruits and vegetables, someday will be known all over the world." And that's exactly what happened. My father's recovery gave birth to the most wonderful product line of fruit and vegetable concentrates, Juice Plus+®.

My father taught me pride and honor. He would tell me that a man's word is all he has. In more than 50 years of being a carpenter, he never once had a written contract with anyone—only an agreement of a smile, honor, and love. He will always own a piece of my heart. I know he is always with me; he's my strength and motivation.

Juice Plus+® Formulation

The two original Juice Plus+® formulas are the Garden Blend® and the Orchard Blend®, which jointly contain natural powders from 15 different fruits and vegetables and bran from two grains, as listed below. The powders are concentrated from the juice and pulp of the fruits and vegetables using a proprietary process that retains more of the original nutrition than standard fruit and vegetable processing.

Juice Plus+ Garden Blend®	**Juice Plus+ Orchard Blend®**
Beet	Acerola cherry
Broccoli	Apple
Cabbage	Cranberry
Carrot	Orange
Kale	Papaya
Parsley	Peach
Spinach	Pineapple
Tomato	
Oat bran	
Rice bran	

In addition, Juice Plus+® contains digestive enzymes and probiotics; these are detailed in chapter 3. I developed all three Juice Plus+® formulas—the Garden Blend®, Orchard Blend®, and recently the Vineyard Blend® (see chapter 5)—keeping in mind the balance needed for what ultimately became chapter 3's Triad Approach to healing. The Juice Plus+® Foundational Nutrition chart in the next section shows how the specific components of all three formulas work together to benefit different organs.

Juice Plus+® as Foundational Nutrition

To get to the bottom line of nutrition, health, disease, and healing, we must always consider both the physical and energetic aspects of our bodies and the foods and supplements we consume. Furthermore, because everything in the body is connected, and the whole body is involved in all health conditions, it's necessary when treating a specific condition to treat the whole body as well—with foundational nutrition. Foundational nutrition helps balance the body's physical and energetic aspects, and acts to enhance the effectiveness of other supplementation while the body heals itself.

Demonstrated benefits. Juice Plus+® is a proven whole-food foundational supplement. The research behind Juice Plus+® (listed below) has shown that it provides bioavailable nutrients;

increases the body's absorption and blood levels of phytochemicals, vitamins, and minerals; supports immune system function; positively affects key indicators of cardiovascular health, including arterial elasticity; and has the antioxidant effects of reducing oxidative stress and protecting DNA from free radical attack.

- *Houston MC et al. Juice powder concentrate and systemic blood pressure, progression of coronary artery calcium and antioxidant status in hypertensive subjects: a pilot study. Evidence-Based Compl Altern Med 2007 doi:10.1093/ecam/nel108*

- *Kawashima A et al. Four week supplementation with mixed fruit and vegetable juice concentrates increased protective serum antioxidants and folate and decreased plasma homocysteine in Japanese subjects. Asia Pacific J Clin Nutr 2007 16:411–421*

- *Bloomer RJ et al. Oxidative stress response to aerobic exercise: comparison of antioxidant supplements. Med Sci Sports Exerc 2006 38:1098–1105*

- *Kiefer L et al. Supplementation with mixed fruit and vegetable juice concentrates increased serum antioxidants and folate in healthy adults. J Am Coll Nutr 2004 23:205–211*

- *Panunzio MF et al. Supplementation with fruit and vegetable concentrate decreases plasma homocysteine in a dietary controlled trial. Nutr Res 2003 23:1221–1228*

- *Plotnick GD et al. Effect of supplemental phytonutrients on impairment of the flow-mediated brachial artery vasoactivity after a single high-fat meal. J Am Coll Cardiol 2003 41:1744–1749*

- *Samman S et al. A mixed fruit and vegetable concentrate increases plasma antioxidant vitamins and folate and lowers plasma homocysteine in men. J Nutr 2003 133:2188–2193*

- *Leeds AR et al. Availability of micronutrients from dried, encapsulated fruit and vegetable preparations: a study in healthy volunteers. J Hum Nutr Dietetics 2000 13:21–27*

- *Inserra PF et al. Immune function in elderly smokers and nonsmokers improves during supplementation with fruit and vegetable extracts. Integr Med 1999 2:3–10*

- *Smith MJ et al. Supplementation with fruit and vegetable extracts may decrease DNA damage in the peripheral lymphocytes of an elderly population. Nutr Res 1999 19:1507–1518*

- *Wise JA et al. Changes in plasma carotenoids, alpha-tocopherol, and lipid peroxide levels in response to supplementation with concentrated fruit and vegetable extracts: a pilot study. Curr Ther Res 1996 57:445–461)*

Acupuncturists and kinesiologists have also discovered that the energy make-up of Juice Plus+® helps support and balance all of the acupuncture meridians. That's how it brings Eastern and Western medicine together, as shown below. This version of chapter 3's Balancing and Healing Chart incorporates most of the ingredients in the three Juice Plus+® blends. You can see here that in addition to the overall effects of Juice Plus+® on the body as a whole, the formulas' specific ingredients also support the energy and activity of specific organs.

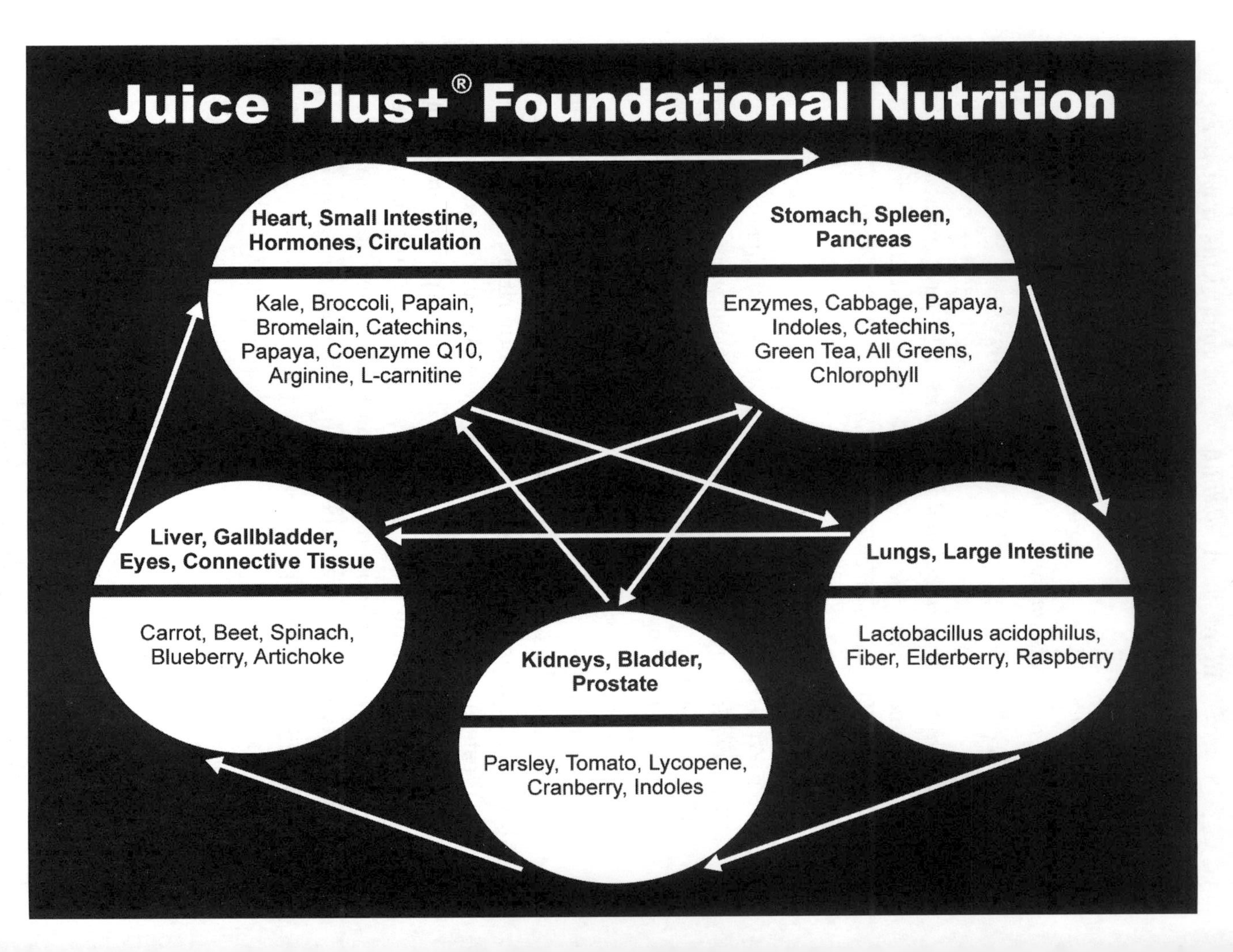
Juice Plus+® Foundational Nutrition
Heart, Small Intestine, Hormones, Circulation
Kale, Broccoli, Papain, Bromelain, Catechins, Papaya, Coenzyme Q10, Arginine, L-carnitine
Stomach, Spleen, Pancreas
Enzymes, Cabbage, Papaya, Indoles, Catechins, Green Tea, All Greens, Chlorophyll
Liver, Gallbladder, Eyes, Connective Tissue
Carrot, Beet, Spinach, Blueberry, Artichoke
Lungs, Large Intestine
Lactobacillus acidophilus, Fiber, Elderberry, Raspberry
Kidneys, Bladder, Prostate
Parsley, Tomato, Lycopene, Cranberry, Indoles

Morning, noon, and night. Everything in nature has a rhythm—night and day, the tides, the menstrual cycle, the seasons... Your organs have an energy rhythm too. Remember the organ clock in chapter 3? Some physicians follow the theory that to strengthen a weak organ, that organ's peak energy period is the best time to administer its supplement or medication.

Fortunately, a foundational supplement taken at any time during the 24-hour period provides general support to all meridians and organs. However, taking Juice Plus+® before, between, or with meals is also helpful to the body at particular parts of the day and into the night:

- Between 5:00 and 7:00 a.m., when the large intestine is most active, it's time to eliminate. The fruit juice powders in the Orchard Blend® assist morning elimination.
- Between 7:00 and 9:00 a.m., with more energy in the stomach, you're ready for breakfast. The Vineyard Blend® helps kick-start your body's functions for the morning.
- As the day progresses, the energies of other organs—pancreas, heart, bladder, kidneys—are dominant in turn. Juice Plus+® assists their activities by causing vasodilation (vessel expansion), thereby increasing blood circulation throughout the body—which has many beneficial effects.
- The bioavailable nutrients in Juice Plus+® can help compensate for things that your day's food may lack. The Orchard Blend® and Vineyard Blend® offer many of the nutrients in fruits and berries, while the Garden Blend® helps offset the vegetable shortage in the typical diet.
- Taken before and after workouts, the Vineyard Blend® improves overall oxygen utilization and toxin elimination. This formula's tissue-specific antioxidants and particular healing virtues are detailed in chapter 5.
- Because of its chlorophyll content, the Garden Blend® taken between meals or at lunch or dinner assists your body's self-cleansing processes. In the evening, a night-long detox cycle begins as the energies of the gallbladder, liver, and lungs become dominant. *Note:* Don't eat at night,

because that'll throw your body into a digestive cycle, inhibiting detoxification and waste elimination.

Energy Medicine and Foundational Nutrition

You've now learned that all bodily organs, functions, and secretions are connected energetically, in parallel with physiological connections and pathological processes. The body's physical and energetic aspects are not really separate; they are one and the same, because the physical body in reality *is* energy. It's just that we can see the body, but not the invisible energy circulating through it—as we can see a light bulb, but not the energy that produces its glow, and yet that energy exists.

The arrows of the energy cycles on the chart also demonstrate pathology, "the path which disease travels." As symptoms manifest, they move along the body's energy pathways. When we look at symptoms and sicknesses, we know that the physical symptoms are actually the energies of the body expressing themselves. When the energies and meridians are balanced, the restoration of the physical body quickly follows.

Energy and healing. Is it so far-fetched to conceive of the physical body as an energy manifestation? This truth unites all healing arts. To diagnose is to recognize the expression of nature within. No matter what type of therapy is used, the body heals itself—what we're doing with any treatment is trying to bring the body back into balance by giving it what it needs to heal.

Because the body is an energy manifestation, the electrical characteristics of heartbeats can be measured with an electrocardiogram (EKG) to diagnose abnormalities of heart activity—this is energy medicine. An electroencephalogram (EEG) can be used to detect abnormalities in the brain's electrical activity—also energy medicine. All healing professionals, in fact, use energy medicine, whether they know it or admit it.

No one can be an expert in all healing modalities. But we all need foundational nutrition, so one thing is certain: in their use of energy medicine, all physicians and other health practitioners can and should use foundational supplementation with their patients, especially while working on elderly people.

The acupuncturist. Acupuncture was one of the first uses of energy medicine. The acupuncturist's objective is to balance the meridians and restore proper energy flow so healing can occur. To treat an energy imbalance or blockage, tiny, hair-thin needles are placed in several points, each connected energetically to a specific body part or process. The needles draw energy to those points to balance the flow, so the body can then heal itself.

You could have knee pain because of blockage in the kidney meridian, which flows from the bottom of the feet up the legs, but not know the real cause unless you go to an acupuncturist. The acupuncturist can treat the blockage and the pain, while administering foundational nutritional supplementation that supports the whole body to increase its healing energies.

The chiropractor. When vertebrae or other joints are out of alignment, they can impinge upon nerves, and the resulting blockage of nerve energy causes energy deficiency in the organs and tissues along the affected pathway. This deficiency leads those areas to accumulate excessive metabolic waste, reducing their nutritional status—which can start a chain reaction of impairment throughout the body's energetic interconnections.

When the chiropractor adjusts (realigns) the vertebrae, the blocked energy from the spine is released through the nervous system. Administering foundational supplementation enhances the effectiveness of chiropractic treatment by supporting the flow of that energy to the affected areas and all other meridians. More specific supplements can be used after the adjustment.

The medical doctor. Despite their use of energy medicine through various diagnostic and treatment tools, conventional doctors don't talk about meridians, Chinese medicine, or foundational nutrition in their approach to healing—but I'm drawing the connection between Eastern and Western medicine to show their commonalities. We're really all on the same path.

The medical doctor usually treats one or more of the sick patient's primary symptoms, but a health problem affects all bodily systems. In conjunction with the doctor's specific therapies, foundational supplementation can support the whole body. This holistic approach helps prevent overstimulation of some organs and weakening of others during treatment.

The dietitian, nutritionist, and naturopath. These healers use herbal and nutritional supplementation for deficiencies, balancing, and cleansing. Most supplements act on specific body parts or tissues, and most have both primary and secondary actions, whether they're being used to fight infection, cleanse an organ, add "insurance" to the diet, or support athletic activity.

In my years of practicing herbology and nutrition, I've found that over-supplementation—aside from being expensive—can overwork an organ, which can then deplete or overstimulate another one. A heavy supplement regimen can overtax the liver, and as its energy decreases, digestion gets worse too. This is a major stress on an already sick body, as it takes a lot of energy to metabolize massive amounts of supplements. Energy imbalance further weakens patients, especially the chronically ill.

Each organ system has to keep up with the pace of the others. You can't do a whole lot of bowel cleansing, for example, without affecting the kidneys or spleen. So it makes sense, while focusing on a specific organ or system, to support them all with foundational supplementation. And with this approach, you don't always have to give your clients 15 different formulas.

The homeopath. Homeopathy was probably the first form of vibrational medicine. "Like cures like" is the theory. Before the 1900s, most of the medications used in this country were homeopathic, typically a dilution of whatever substance was thought to be causing the patient's problem. It was later discovered that harmful entities such as toxic chemicals, heavy metals, bacteria, viruses, and parasites could be removed from the body by using a vibrational source giving off the exact same frequency as the entity's, but greatly magnified or potentized.

Homeopathic remedies are now prepared by specialized equipment that potentizes and imprints vibrations in the full spectrum useful for combating microorganisms and detoxifying, toning, and rebuilding tissues. For example, to make a remedy for a staph infection, a culture of the bacteria is placed on the instrument's input plate, and its greatly magnified vibrations are imprinted on a solution of water and alcohol on the output plate. When taken, the remedy's emanating vibrations spread through the body and kill the staph bacteria.

Along with remedies, homeopaths now use herbal, vitamin, and mineral supplements for mutual enhancement of their activities. In my practice, I've found that supporting the body with foundational nutrition while giving homeopathic remedies yields better results. Homeopathy can be combined with any other therapy, often very effectively. For example, in hormone replacement therapy, taking a hormone or glandular product with its corresponding potentized remedy speeds the process.

The kinesiologist. Clinical kinesiology, based on Chinese acupuncture philosophy, has been widely used for the past 40 years. It monitors the energetics of the body by testing the responses of the muscles that have been found to relate to specific meridians and organs. If stress, toxins, deficiencies, infections, and such are blocking energy in the body, the muscle testing will identify the affected area(s). The kinesiologist then utilizes supplements or other methods to strengthen those areas. This form of diagnosis and healing depends on the individual's unique energy feedback system—definitely energy medicine! And again, foundational nutrition is of paramount importance to support all systems while working on specific problems.

The electral dermal screening (EDS) and bio-resonance practitioner. These advanced, complicated methods have been used in Germany for more than 60 years. In brief, the energy feedback from acupuncture points is read by a tiny probe attached to a computer. A knowledgeable practitioner can not only test every function, hormone, nutrient, or disease in the body, but can also make a remedy with the specific energetic frequency—chosen from thousands of herbal and homeopathic resonances—to correct the imbalance or treat the condition.

The presence of toxins, infection, hormone imbalance, genetic problems, effects of past vaccinations, and mental or physical stress can be assessed in moments. Clinicians using this type of energy medicine balance all the meridians and create personalized healing programs, including remedies for past and present emotional traumas. These practitioners understand the importance of foundational supplementation in conjunction with other therapies, and they love Juice Plus+®, saying it reduces the amount of supplements their clients have to take.

The massage therapist. Deep tissue massage stimulates acupuncture points, meridians, and blood and lymph flow. Lymphatic and blood circulation carry nutrients and wastes to and from all organs and systems. So the liver had better be able to process the accumulated toxins stimulated by massage to move through the body, and the bowels had better be in good working condition to expel them—moving poisons around without eliminating them properly can have drastic effects. Insightful massage therapists understand this and use supplementation to enhance detoxification. A little knowledge of foundational nutrition goes a long way here.

Chapter 5
Juice Plus+ Vineyard Blend®: Why It Works

It's the intelligence within the body that heals, but we must supply it with supportive nutrients so healing and rebuilding can happen. My first two Juice Plus+® formulas, the Garden Blend® and Orchard Blend® (detailed in chapter 4), were the focus of most of the initial research studies and should be used as the baseline of your foundational nutrition program.

My latest formula, the Juice Plus+ Vineyard Blend®, features juice powder from grapes and berries, along with enzymes and several other special ingredients. We greatly need such a supplement as an antioxidant source, and especially because berries are a missing link in preventing today's epidemic of cardiovascular disease. Isn't it interesting that the very foods now missing in our diets are the ones that can prevent our primary ailments? Berries were a part of mankind's sustenance for thousands of years. I guess we just forgot!

What makes any whole food work, nutritionally speaking, is its thousands of phytochemicals, also called phytonutrients. Many have been identified and studied, and many are yet to be discovered. The totality of a food's phytonutrients produces its synergistic effects. But nowadays, even our whole foods are often nutrient-deficient. Supplements are therefore a necessity in today's living experience—especially if you're sick or weak or your digestion is not working properly. For complete health, optimal function, and healing, using a whole-food concentrate such as Juice Plus+® to supplement your spectrum of nutrients may be your best bet.

A Note on Primary Research

You can't simply throw foods, herbs, vitamins, and minerals into a capsule without regard for their interactions and effects on each other. Many individual herbs are terrific for the heart, for example, but if combined in the wrong ratio or mixture, they may be minimally helpful or not at all.

In developing a combination formula, there are several considerations: the nutrients in the ingredients, their physical and energetic compatibility, the ratio that will prevent any substances from dominating or competing for absorption, and whether the nutrients will be broken down or used up before they can get to the tissues and functions they're intended to support. What is the bioactivity of the combined substances? Will the body's cells recognize the formula's "cellular identity"?

Of basic importance in addressing those formulating considerations is primary research conducted on the combined formula—not "borrowed" research conducted on the separate ingredients. Unfortunately, few companies are willing to spend the money, and many inadequately researched combinations are on the market. NSA, however, has done nothing but primary research on each Juice Plus+® formula (see the references in chapter 4). The ratio of foods, the enzymatic activity, the energetics of each ingredient, and the techniques of its manufacture make the Vineyard Blend® a stand-alone product.

Virtues of the Vineyard

You might have heard such scientific terms as carotenoids, flavanols, tannins, polyphenols, anthocyanins, and others even more difficult to pronounce. These and other phytochemicals are named and categorized according to their distinct characteristics, activities, and effects on our metabolism or tissues. The pigments in foods are actually some of the phytonutrients most important for our health—I think it's so interesting that colors help the body heal itself!

The overall effects of the Vineyard Blend® are increased blood flow, improved oxygen supply to the tissues, enhanced waste elimination, increased absorption of other supplements, and helping to prevent heart disease. Furthermore, each ingredient has specific health effects. Bilberry, for example, increases circulation, and elderberry decongests the sinuses and lungs. But I'm not saying that bilberries cure circulatory problems or that elderberries cure lung problems, because they don't—the body speaks, the body heals. All Juice Plus+® formulas include a variety of whole foods and other ingredients so the healing power within the body can pick what it needs.

Bilberry. Bilberry has more than 100 identified constituents, including potent antioxidants. It's been used in ophthalmologic, peripheral vascular, and venous circulation conditions, with studies conducted mainly in ophthalmology and vascular insufficiency. Bilberry demonstrates protection against capillary fragility and diabetic retinopathy, helps decrease early signs of capillary inflammation, reduces bruising, and may decrease retinal damage. *(Muth ER et al. The effect of bilberry supplementation on night visual acuity and contrast sensitivity. Altern Med Rev 2000 5:164–173; Morazzoni P, Bombardelli E. Vaccinium myrtillus L. Fitoterapia 1996 67:3–29; Grieve MA. A Modern Herbal. Jonathan Cape Ltd., London, UK, 1931)*

Cranberry. Cranberry's anthocyanins inhibit bacteria from adhering to and penetrating the mucosal wall of the kidneys, bladder, and urinary tract. In one study, women given cranberry juice had 42 percent fewer urinary tract infections (UTIs) than the placebo group. (*Escherichia coli* bacteria cause 80–90 percent of UTIs.) The berry's quinic acid also helps prevent kidney stone formation. And compared to broccoli, cranberry has five times as much of the antioxidants that inhibit development of atherosclerosis, cancer, and other degenerative diseases. *(Howell AB, Foxman B. Cranberry juice and adhesion of antibiotic-resistant uropathogens. JAMA 2002 287:3082–3083; Vinson JA et al. Phenol antioxidant quantity and quality in foods: fruits. J Agric Food Chem 2001 49:5315–5321)*

Elderberry. Elderberry increases circulation to the lungs and heart and decreases congestion in lungs and swollen joints. It contains vitamins A, B, and C, as well as the anti-inflammatory antioxidants quercetin and rutin. *(Milbury PE et al. Bioavailability of elderberry anthocyanins. Mech Ageing Dev 2002 123:997–1006; Wu X, Prior R. Absorption and metabolism of anthocyanins in elderly women after consumption of elderberry or blueberry. J Nutr 2002 132:1865–1871; Leitner G et al. Stress induced electrolyte and blood gas changes with and without a six days oral treatment with* *elderberry (Sambucus nigra L.) concentrate. Magnesium Bull 2000 22:72–76; Abuja PM et al. Antioxidant and prooxidant activities of elderberry (Sambucus nigra) extract in low-density lipoprotein oxidation. J Agric Food Chem 1998 46:4091–4096)*

Black currant. Black currants contain strong antioxidants and are very nutritious, boasting three times the amount of vitamin C in oranges, along with iron, magnesium, phosphorus, potassium, vitamins B_1, B_2, B_3, and B_5, and zinc.

This berry also has an important relationship with the brain. By inhibiting the enzyme monoamine oxidase (MAO), which is a natural regulator of neurotransmitter levels, a patented black currant extract has been shown to activate the brain and central nervous system. It has a pronounced effect on dopamine, a neurotransmitter involved in functions including testosterone balance and modulation of mood and cerebral performance. This has exciting implications for preventing and treating neurodegenerative disorders associated with reduced cerebral performance, such as Parkinson's disease, dementia, and mood disorders. In Parkinson's, black currant extract has inhibited further degeneration of dopamine neuron receptors. *(Erlund I et al. Consumption of black currants, lingonberries and bilberries increases serum quercetin concentrations. Eur J Clin Nutr 2003 57:37–42; Nakaishi H et al. Effects of black currant anthocyanoside intake on dark adaptation and VDT-work-induced transient refractive alteration in healthy humans. Altern Med Rev 2000 5:553–56; Bormann J et al. Use of blackcurrant juice to promote monoamine oxidase inhibition for increasing cerebral performance, treating and preventing Parkinson's disease, etc. US Patent 91755814, 1991; see also red currant citations, below)*

Red currant. Closely related to black currant, red currant has less of their shared constituents, but provides antioxidants and is high in magnesium, vitamins B_1, B_2, B_3, and C, and zinc. English and German research sources consider this berry to be astringent, a digestive aid, fever reducing, and menstruation inducing. It's used for connective tissue disease, fibromyalgia, gout, and rheumatism. Red currant is an antiseptic for the lungs and sinuses and can also act as a blood cleanser and diuretic.

(Beattie J et al. Potential health benefits of berries. Curr Nutr Food Sci 2005 1:71–86; Kahkonen MP et al. Berry phenolics and their antioxidant activity. J Agric Food Chem 2001 49:4076–4082)

Blueberry. Highest in antioxidants in a study of 40 fruits and vegetables, this berry exhibits a remarkable variety of effects. Reports state that eating blueberries can counteract free radical damage to the arteries and even reverse it in the central nervous system. In addition to UTI-preventive compounds, blueberry also contains phytonutrients that improve cell membrane fluidity, allowing nutrients and chemical signals to pass in and out of cells and reducing inflammatory processes.

Exciting research indicates that blueberry can ameliorate age-related neural and cognitive declines in neurodegenerative disorders such as Alzheimer's disease, and has potential for reversing age-related balance, motor coordination, and memory impairment. Other studies show improvements in dopamine release, eye weakness, and liver function. *(Schmidt BM et al. Effective separation of potent antiproliferation and antiadhesion components from wild blueberry (Vaccinium angustifolium Ait.) fruits. J Agric Food Chem 2004 52:6433–6442; Joseph JA et al. Reversals of age-related declines in neuronal signal transduction, cognitive, and motor behavioral deficits with blueberry, spinach, or strawberry dietary supplementation. J Neuroscience 1999 19:8114–8121; Prior RL et al. Antioxidant capacity as influenced by total phenolic and anthocyanin content, maturity, and variety of Vaccinium species. J Agric Food Chem 1998 46:2686–2693)*

Raspberry. This berry's nutritional profile is tremendous: calcium, carotenes, magnesium, manganese, potassium, salicylic acid, quercetin, and vitamins B_5, C, and E. Raspberry also has 4–6 grams of fiber per 100 grams, more than apple, banana, and pear. Most important is its high content of ellagic acid, an antibacterial nutrient that promotes carcinogen detoxification; in one study, ellagic acid was found to block various hormonal reactions and metabolic pathways associated with cancer development. Raspberry has been shown to slow the growth of abnormal colon cells, prevent the development of cells infected with human papilloma virus (HPV) linked to cervical cancer, and trigger natural death of prostate cancer cells. *(EA Decker. The role of phenolics, conjugated linoleic acid, carnosine, and pyrroloquinoline quinone as nonessential dietary antioxidants. Nutr Rev 1995 53:49–58; Maas JL et al. Evaluation of strawberry genotypes for ellagic acid, an antimutagenic and anticarcinogenic plant phenol. In: The Strawberry into the 21st Century. A Dale and JJ Luby, eds. Timber Press, Portland, OR, 1991; Jones KC, Klocke JA. Aphid feeding deterrence of ellagitannins, their phenolic hydrolysis products and related phenolic derivatives. Entomol Expt Appl 1987 44:229–234)*

Blackberry. Known for its content of ellagic acid (see above), fiber, minerals, and quercetin, blackberry also boasts beta carotene, folic acid, lutein, vitamins C and K, and zeaxanthin—phytonutrients especially good for the eyes. Its tannins are thought to underlie its astringent action against loose bowels and dysentery. Blackberry is posited to benefit the liver and to strengthen the heart when kidney problems are present. Its oxygen radical absorbance capacity (ORAC), a measure of antioxidant ability, is one of the highest of all fruits: 5,347 per 100 grams. *(Hager TJ et al. Ellagitannin composition of blackberry as determined by HPLC-ESI-MS and MALDI-TOF-MS. J Agric Food Chem 2008 56:661–669; Grieve MA. A Modern Herbal. Jonathan Cape Ltd., London, UK, 1931)*

Concord grape. Grape's quercetin blocks the histamine-initiated inflammatory cascade in allergies, arthritis, and fibromyalgia. Quercetin and catechins, a bioflavonoid subgroup, are responsible for grape's strong antioxidant capacity, with far-reaching effects against oxidative damage to proteins and fats.

Intact proteins and fats are needed for hormonal balance, immune system actions, and many other functions. Low-density lipoproteins (LDLs), for example, carry needed fats to tissues for use in cell membranes. But when free radicals oxidize LDLs, their fats turn rancid, so the membranes harden, nutrients can't get in, fluids escape, and cells die. In the bloodstream, oxidized LDLs form arterial plaque, reducing oxygenation and blood flow and leading to heart disease. Antioxidants to the rescue! Blood levels of free radicals dropped 20 percent in study participants taking vitamin E or Concord grape juice daily for two weeks—but only the grape juice group had a 20 percent reduction in oxidation-damaged proteins, a finding with huge implications for fat metabolism and heart disease prevention. *(O'Byrne DJ et al. Comparison of the antioxidant effects of Concord grape juice flavonoids and alpha-tocopherol on markers of oxidative stress in healthy adults. Am J Clin Nutr 2002 76:1367–1374)*

Green tea. Green tea's polyphenols are bioflavonoids, a group of more than 4,000 compounds that are powerful antioxidants, can be helpful against many health conditions, (particularly heart disease), and may modify the body's reaction to allergens, carcinogens, and viruses.

Stronger antioxidants than vitamins C and E, green tea phytonutrients have been proven to help neutralize toxins in the intestines, liver, and lungs. They seem to trap, and inhibit the formation of, cancer-causing agents. In studies of breast cancer cells, green tea extract inhibited their growth. Population studies indicate that green tea consumption may be a main reason for Japan's low cancer rate. *(Komori A et al. Anticarcinogenic activity of green tea polyphenols. Jap J Clin Oncol 1993 23:186–190; Katiyar SK et al. Green tea in chemoprevention of cancer. Compr Ther 1992 18:3–8; Mukhtar H et al. Tea components: antimutagenic and anticarcinogenic effects. Prev Med 1992 21:351–360)*

Grape seed extract. Grape seed contains procyanidolic oligomers (PCOs), bioflavonoids first used decades ago for blood vessel disorders. Although vitamin E inhibits the LDL oxidation that's a key factor in artery hardening and heart disease, it's outdone by these PCOs—50 times more potent an antioxidant, and they prevent platelet clumping that can lead to blood clots and strokes.

Connective tissue gives you flexibility and youthful skin and holds you together. Free radical damage to this tissue causes degenerative joint disease and other inflammatory conditions. Grape seed PCOs bind to its collagen and elastin, protecting against oxidation, painful swelling, and inflammatory damage. PCOs are also antihistaminic and anti-allergic; they block the enzyme hyaluronidase (which causes inflammation via histamine release) and reduce histamine's production and effect.

(Facino RM et al. Free radicals scavenging action and anti-enzyme activities of procyanidines from Vitis vinifera: a mechanism for their capillary protective action. Arzneimittelforschung 1994 44:592–601; Jialal I, Grundy SM. Effect of combined supplementation with alpha-tocopherol ascorbate and beta-carotene on low-density lipoprotein oxidation. Circulation 1993 88:2780–2786; Schwitters B, Masquelier J. OPC in Practice: Biflavanols and Their Application. Alfa Amega, Rome, Italy, 1993)

Ginger. This herb has traditional uses in Chinese medicine and acts as a carrier for other substances in combination formulas. A known vasodilator, ginger is also known to increase the stomach's secretions and stimulate the digestive tract, working very well along with digestive enzymes (see below). Ginger was added to the Vineyard Blend® to promote digestion, increase circulation, and assist in the distribution of nutrients. *(Lu HC. Chinese Natural Cures: Traditional Methods for Remedy and Prevention. Black Dog & Leventhal Publishers, NY, 2006)*

Digestive enzymes. I can't overemphasize good digestion as the first line of health defense. If food isn't digested properly, you won't absorb all of its nutrients, and it ferments in your intestine, producing toxins that can be reabsorbed into the lymphatic system and bloodstream. To aid digestion and the elimination of toxic colon buildup, the Vineyard Blend® contains the four main enzyme groups described in chapter 3: protease, amylase, lipase, and cellulase. For more information, see my books *Food Enzymes: The Missing Link to Radiant Health (Hohm Press, Prescott, AZ, 1993)* and *ProMetabolics: Your Personal Guide to Transformational Health and Healing (Designs for Wellness Press, Carlsbad, CA, 2008).*

Proteolytic enzymes. These enzymes are critical to the blood's constant interaction of clotting and clot-dissolving. In response to cell damage, clots of fibrin protein seal off the damaged area—but obstructed blood flow increases swelling and inflammation, so the fibrin must be dissolved to let fresh oxygenated blood in, or pain, heat, and swelling will persist. Free-radical-induced clotting can thicken arterial walls, reducing blood flow and increasing the risk of a sudden embolism (blockage). Blood cells produce proteolytic enzymes to split fibrin—but if the breakdown is insufficient, too much fibrin leads to "blood stickiness," scar tissue, plaque deposits, impaired circulation, heart disease, and more inflammation.

Degenerative diseases are characterized by inflammation, so enzymes are crucial to help keep it in check—but as we age, we become enzyme-deficient. Proteolytic enzymes in foods break up clots and also activate the blood's proteolytic system. Large doses are used worldwide for sports injuries and after surgery. The Vineyard Blend® contains a maintenance dose of papain (from papaya) and bromelain (from pineapple), which work with bioflavonoids and vitamin C—and berries are loaded with those, so this formula is a tremendous support against circulatory disease. *(Loomis HF. Enzymes: The Key to Health, Vol. 1. 21st Century Publishing, Madison, WI, 1999; Cichoke AJ. Enzymes and Enzyme Therapy. Keats Publishing, New Canaan, CT, 1994)*

L-carnitine. L-carnitine plays a crucial role in bringing long-chain fatty acids into cells' mitochondria to be burned for energy. Elevated blood levels of cholesterol and other fats have many negative effects, including inhibiting certain immune system functions; l-carnitine helps counteract these effects by removing fats from the blood for cellular metabolism, particularly by the muscles and central nervous system.

L-carnitine deficiency leads to impaired energy metabolism, fatigue, and decreased bone mass, with weight gain a likely result. Some l-carnitine is synthesized in the body, but it's mostly obtained from food, primarily meat and dairy; other sources include nuts, seeds, legumes, certain vegetables and fruits and grains, bee pollen, carob—and the Vineyard Blend®.

By promoting the use of fat for energy and thereby minimizing muscle protein breakdown, l-carnitine taken before workouts enhances exercise capacity, performance, and lean muscle production. It can also improve cardiac function in congestive heart failure; one six-month study demonstrated a 26 percent increase in exercise time and a 14 percent increase in blood pumped in one stroke. *(Mancini M et al. Controlled study on the therapeutic efficacy of propionyl-l-carnitine in patients with congestive heart failure. Arzneimittelforschung 1992 42:1101–1104; Fain JN. Biochemical aspects of drug and hormone action on adipose tissue. Pharmacol Rev 1973 25:67–118)*

Arginine. Although classified as a non-essential amino acid, arginine is absolutely essential for wound healing, and quickly goes to work to repair any injured tissue. Many athletes are familiar with arginine, as it also stimulates the pituitary gland to release growth hormone—see chapter 6—and helps burn fat, tone muscle, and improve performance and physique. *(Fried R, Merrell W. The Arginine Solution. Warner Books, NY, 1999)*

Coenzyme Q10 (CoQ10). Every cell in the body needs CoQ10, the "ignition of the cell," to produce energy. It functions in the cellular manufacture of adenosine triphosphate (ATP) to stimulate metabolic processes. With a CoQ10 deficiency, the cellular engine misfires and fatigue results. Severe deficiency causes engine failure: no ignition, no energy, no life. CoQ10 is also a potent antioxidant and boosts the immune system's disease-fighting capabilities. Studies have shown its vital role in preventing and treating many major diseases (see the appendix). *(Stocker R. Possible health benefits of coenzyme Q10. Linus Pauling Inst Sci Med Newsletter Fall/Winter 2002; Folkers K et al. The activities of coenzyme Q10 and vitamin B6 for immune responses. Biochem Biophys Res Commun 1993 193:88–92)*

Artichoke. Similarly to milk thistle, artichoke extract protects the liver from toxins. It helps regenerate liver cells, and over weeks of use has significantly restored severely damaged livers. Artichoke extract reduces bloodstream levels of cholesterol and other fats by mobilizing them for excretion from the body. Research has focused on its use in preventing atherosclerosis. Artichoke extract has also been used for digestive and gallbladder problems and jaundice. *(Eberhardt G. Untersuchungen ueber die wirkung von cynabei leberzellvertettung. Z Gastroenterol 1973 11:183; Hammerl H et al. Ueber den einfluss von cynarin auf hyperlipidaemien untr besonderer beruechsichtingung des typs II (hypercholesterinaemie). Wiener Medizinische Wochenschrift 1973 41:601; Greten H et al. Die lipoproteinelektrophorese zur diagnose von hyperlipoproteinaemian. Deutsche Medizinische Wochenschrift 1970*

95:1716; Caruzzo C et al. Considerazioni sull'attivita dell'acido 1,4-dicaffeilchinoco sulle frzioni lipidiche del siero nell'aterosclerosi. Minerva Med 1969 60:4514)

Antioxidants and Anti-Aging

I'm sure you noticed that many of the constituents in the Vineyard Blend®'s ingredients are antioxidants. Why is this so important? Because free radical damage and oxidative stress are linked to the aging process and to countless health conditions, including all chronic diseases, inflammatory diseases, and diseases of aging.

A destructive chain. Anywhere in the body, any molecule that loses an electron becomes an unstable free radical, which must then steal an electron from another molecule to rebalance itself—creating another free radical. It's estimated that each of our cells gets "hit" by a free radical 100,000 times a day. Membranes, enzymes, proteins, hormones, neurotransmitters, nutrients, and the like are damaged when electrons are stolen from them, weakening tissues and organs and interfering with countless necessary functions. When free radicals damage a cell's DNA, genetic mutation can result.

Free radical damage and oxidative stress occur every second in your body. Ironically, a significant amount is due to natural cellular activities. Anything that causes cells to use oxygen, including their normal metabolic and physiological processes, produces free radicals. Free radicals are also created by environmental pollution, smoking, fried and processed food, and any kind of physical stress—including exercise. Through poor eating and health habits that actually speed up free radical production, we contribute even more to our own premature, accelerated aging and systemic inflammation.

Oxidation, inflammation, aging, and disease. If free radicals are overabundant and the resulting oxidative stress in the body is not controlled, a consequence is inflammation. One form of oxidative stress is the lipid peroxidation that turns fat rancid, damaging fat-containing substances and membranes.

The brain, being more than 60 percent fat, is particularly vulnerable to this damage, which is related to dementia and neurological disorders such as Parkinson's and Alzheimer's. Free radical damage to the brain and its "master controllers"—the hypothalamus, pineal gland, and pituitary gland—can lead to hormonal imbalance and chronic inflammation. Other factors contributing to inflammation include heavy metal toxicity, decreased oxygen to the brain, and nutritional deficiencies.

Most of us have some kind of inflammation going on somewhere, though we may not know it. When the immune system must constantly battle inflammation, the body becomes fatigued, weakened, and deficient in nutrients and enzymes. And the more inflammation damages your arterial walls, heart, lungs, joints, and brain, the faster you age. Inflammation also contributes to all degenerative diseases, especially arthritis and autoimmune disorders.

During chronic inflammation, hormones called cytokines are at high levels and can cause the body to attack itself. The cytokine interleukin-6 is abnormally high in Alzheimer's, atherosclerosis, cancer, osteoporosis, and rheumatoid arthritis. Cytokine levels rise with age as well. As cytokines increase, the hormone dehydroepiandrosterone (DHEA) decreases. Research shows that declining DHEA can contribute to neurological diseases, anxiety, and loss of libido. Fortunately, supplemental DHEA can come to the rescue (see the appendix). *(Null G. Power Aging. New American Library, NY, 2003; Genazzani AD et al. Oral dehydroepiandrosterone supplementation modulates spontaneous and growth hormone-releasing hormone-induced growth hormone and insulin-like growth factor-1 secretion in early and late postmenopausal women. Fertil Steril 2001 76:241–248; Cutolo M. Sex hormone adjuvant therapy in rheumatoid arthritis. Rheum Dis Clin North Am 2000 26:881–895; Arlt W et al. Dehydroepiandrosterone replacement in women with adrenal insufficiency. N Engl J Med 1999 341:1013–1020; Bellino FL et al. DHEA and aging. Aging 1995 774:1–350)*

The antidotes. Oxidative stress and inflammation are preventable epidemics. What is your defense? To protect your brain and body from free radical damage, inflammation, and age-related health conditions, you need to increase your consumption of whole foods and whole-food supplements—such as Juice Plus+ Vineyard Blend®—that neutralize free radicals with antioxidant nutrients. Vitamins C and E, many minerals, bioflavonoids, and countless other phytonutrients are natural antioxidants. Fruits and vegetables are loaded with them. All berries are packed full of them. You also need to detoxify and to get your hormones back in balance (see chapter 6). There is no other way! *(Papas AM. Antioxidant Status, Diet, Nutrition, and Health. CRC Press, Boca Raton, FL, 1999; Borek C. Maximize Your Health-Span with Antioxidants. Keats Publishing, New Canaan, CT, 1995)*

Chapter 6
Help for Hormonal Difficulties: Men and Women

Health problems in circle V of chapter 3's Balancing and Healing Chart—heart, circulation, and hormones—are usually a long time in coming, and are a sign that more work has to be done. The likely underlying causes are nutritional deficiencies, years of accumulated toxins, and energetic imbalance. If these are hindering your glands and disturbing your hormonal output, your endocrine system needs support.

This chapter presents specific therapeutic programs for gland support and hormonal balancing through the use of Triad Healing formulas, detoxification, foundational nutrition, and additional specific supplements. And as always, helping the body to regulate any function involves enhancing digestion.

Note: If you're working primarily with another organ or bodily function, but you also have a hormonal imbalance, it's very important to support your endocrine system as well. An inexperienced therapist, however, can mistakenly overlook this—for instance, putting a patient with a hormone issue on a detox program without endocrine support. In such a case, the poisons released into the bloodstream as the patient detoxifies can travel to the already out-of-whack glands and overstimulate them, so the glands work harder, and their increased output further disrupts the existing imbalance and may cause more problems. The moral of this story: don't forget your glands!

Brain, Glands, and Hormones

To understand how to nourish and balance this complex and multifaceted system, you must learn a bit about how it works. No need to memorize anything in this section, though—it's simply intended as an introduction to several of the major players, their interconnections, and some of their functions.

Your endocrine system, from top to bottom, starts in your brain, with the pineal gland, hypothalamus, and pituitary gland;

continues downward, with the thyroid, parathyroid, thymus, and adrenal glands; includes the pancreas and some other organs; and ends at the sex glands. These all work together in a beautiful symphony of interrelated functions—unless one or more parts start playing the wrong notes.

Neurohormones. Neurotransmission is the main way the nervous system communicates, enabling the various parts of the brain to work in harmony. Energy bursts travel along neurons (nerve cells) electrochemically, combining and recombining in reactions and counter-reactions. That energy information is carried across the gaps between neurons by chemicals called neurotransmitters, which are sucked up into the neuron terminals. Of the dozens of neurotransmitters, some have excitatory effects on nerves and brain structures, and others are inhibitory. A balance between excitatory and inhibitory must be maintained to avoid either overstimulation or under-activity.

Given that several brain structures are parts of the endocrine system, it makes sense that certain substances released by specialized neurons can serve as neurohormones; that is, as both neurotransmitters and hormones, depending on where they're acting in the brain or in the body. Examples of neurohormones that you may have heard of include acetylcholine, dopamine, endorphins, epinephrine, melatonin, and serotonin.

Given its different action sites, it also makes sense that a neurohormone can have several functions or effects. A good example is serotonin, which relieves anxiety, panic, and depression, and promotes calmness, relaxation, confidence, and feelings of well-being—and helps regulate intestinal peristalsis. Serotonin also stimulates the adrenals to secrete the hormone aldosterone, causing the kidneys to retain more water and sodium, which increases blood volume and pressure.

Pineal regulation and rhythms. Serotonin is converted to melatonin by the pea-sized pineal gland at the center of the brain. This conversion typically declines with age, which can be a problem, because pineal regulation of the sleep/wake cycle and other circadian rhythms is related to a proper balance between those two neurohormones. Melatonin, nicknamed "the hormone of darkness," is mostly secreted at night, and one of its main functions is to promote sleep; that's why supplemental melatonin and the amino acid tryptophan—a serotonin precursor—are used to combat insomnia. *(Rozencwaig R. The Melatonin and Aging Sourcebook. Hohm Press, Prescott, AZ, 1997)*

Helping the hypothalamus. This almond-sized nerve center above the brain stem is involved in numerous endocrine and other functions. Its acetylcholine, for example, is crucial for the excitatory aspect of the sex drive, helps brain cells communicate with each other, and plays an important role in learning and memory, especially short-term. Acetylcholine metabolism in the brain is maintained by the amino acid derivative acetyl-l-carnitine, which also influences dopamine levels and prevents peroxidation of brain lipids. Supplemental acetyl-l-carnitine is a potent strategy to preserve sexuality and brain function; studies show that 1,000–2,000 milligrams daily can restore a great deal of function to patients with dementia. *(Pettigrew JS et al. Clinical and neurochemical effect of acetyl-l-carnitine in Alzheimer's disease. Neurobiol Aging 1995 16:1–4; Salvioli NM. L-acetyl carnitine in treatment of mental decline in the elderly. Drugs Exptl Clin Res 1994 20:169–176; Sershen H et al. Effect of acetyl-l-carnitine on the dopaminergic system in aging brain. J Neurosci Res 1991 30:555–559)*

Pituitary power. At the base of the brain, this barely marble-sized "master gland" produces a wide variety of hormones to influence all of the other glands and countless bodily functions. Growth hormone (GH) is a well-known pituitary secretion, released mostly at night. GH breaks down in the liver, becoming insulin-like growth factor (IGF-1), which combines with insulin and travels through the bloodstream. This duo maintains lean muscle growth and release fat from adipose tissue for use as fuel, resulting in weight loss from muscle building and fat burning—so you can see why some bodybuilders use GH and insulin injections. GH normally declines with age, but that isn't inevitable if all is well with your lifestyle and supplementation.

Adrenal and thyroid highs and lows. Through its adrenocorticotropic hormone (ACTH), the pituitary prompts the adrenals to secrete various hormones. You may recognize adrenalin (also called epinephrine) and noradrenalin (norepinephrine), which stimulate the nervous system to prepare for "fight or flight." But too much anxiety and stress can lead to excessive adrenal production and burn out these glands—which causes a host of hormonal and other problems.

Acting as an agent of the hypothalamus, the pituitary exerts control over the thyroid as well. In response to thyrotropin-releasing hormone (TRH) from the hypothalamus, the pituitary releases thyrotropin, also called thyroid-stimulating hormone (TSH), prompting the thyroid to produce thyroxin (T4) and triiodothyronine (T3). Thyroid overactivity, or hyperthyroidism, can cause emotional imbalance and reduce libido—and is a potential result of taking synthetic thyroid hormones. Thyroid underactivity, or hypothyroidism, causes exhaustion, lethargy, and depression, and can also reduce testosterone and sex drive. *(Kidd GS et al. The hypothalamus pituitary-adrenal-testicular axis in thyrotoxicosis. J Clin Endocrin Metab 1979 48:798–801)*

Sex hormones, from brain to gonads and back again. The hypothalamus mediates libido in the brain as well as the manufacture of sex hormones farther down the endocrine line. By secreting gonadotropin-releasing hormone (GnRH), which prompts the release of the following pituitary hormones, the hypothalamus initiates a far-reaching cascade of effects on reproductive and sexual functions:

- In both sexes, ACTH prompts the adrenals to convert the prohormone pregnenolone into small amounts of both male and female sex hormones—chiefly, the precursors dehydroepiandrosterone (DHEA) and androstenedione.
- In both sexes, the gonadotropins or "messenger hormones" are follicle-stimulating hormone (FSH) and luteinizing hormone (LH). FSH is important in the female's ovulatory cycle and egg maturation, and stimulates the male's testes to make sperm. LH triggers the female's ovulation and promotes production of estrogens, progesterone, and testosterone by both the male and female gonads.

- In females, prolactin triggers milk production as well as the ovaries' production of progesterone and estrogens. Estrogen is actually the collective name for a group of closely related hormones: estrone, estradiol, and estriol.
- Finally, going full circle, testosterone—converted to estradiol inside hypothalamic neurons—stimulates the hypothalamus and other brain areas that activate libido.
- But remember prolactin? It also decreases sexual desire and suppresses testosterone. Dopamine, which increases desire, has an inverse relationship with prolactin—if the level of one goes up, the other goes down. So if prolactin's up, dopamine and testosterone are down, and libido's inhibited. Sex is complicated! *(Mooradian AD et al. Biological action of androgens. Endocrin Rev 1987 8:1–28; Persky H et al. The relation of plasma androgen levels to sexual behaviors and attitudes of women. Psychosom Med 1982 44:305–319)*

Endocrine Nutrition

Like any other system, the glands need good nutrition. Hormones and neurotransmitters cannot be manufactured unless their building blocks are readily available. When working with the endocrine system (or other organs), it's always good to use whole foods, herbs, and nutritional supplements to supply precursors for your brain and body to make what they need, without overstimulation by drugs or synthetic hormones. And ensuring effective digestion is key to your success, especially if ongoing digestive problems have led to nutritional deficiencies.

Amino acids. An all-purpose amino acid supplement is often suggested while balancing hormones. Why? You may recall that we can't synthesize, and must therefore ingest, eight "essential" amino acids: isoleucine, leucine, lysine, methionine, phenylalanine, threonine, tryptophan, and valine. These and other amino acids are required for many hormones and neurotransmitters. Phenylalanine is used in making insulin; the thyroid needs tyrosine for thyroxin; and serotonin synthesis requires tryptophan—or its variant, 5-hydroxytryptophan (5-HTP), which can cross the blood brain barrier.

An herbal precursor. Dopamine is of interest to athletes because it's essential for coordination and enhances testosterone activity for increased muscle-building. Dopamine synthesis normally requires conversion of tyrosine to the precursor l-dopa, but there are other natural sources of l-dopa. One is an herb called mucuna, long used in India to treat the motor disorder Parkinson's disease. *(www.ars-grin.gov)* Mucuna is a perfect example of herbal synchrony with the brain and body.

Crucial cholesterol. Another critical endocrine nutrient—believe it or not—is cholesterol. This fat is a vitally important building block in the manufacture of all steroid hormones, including sex hormones. Under the direction of the pituitary, specific cells convert cholesterol into pregnenolone, which you encountered earlier as the precursor of progesterone and DHEA. Progesterone and DHEA are then made into aldosterone, cortisol, and androstenedione—and androstenedione, in turn, serves as the precursor for testosterone and estrogens. Whew!

Identifying and Monitoring Hormonal Issues

What can cause glandular and hormonal imbalance?

- stress
- poor diet
- chronic inflammation
- deficiencies of essential fatty acids
- free radical damage
- alcohol and smoking
- decreased oxygen to the brain
- steroids, birth control pills, and medications
- viral and bacterial infections
- indoor and outdoor air and water pollution
- heavy metal toxicity
- fertilizers, pesticides, fungicides, and herbicides
- food additives

The list could go on and on—and even if we don't know it, these things affect us on a daily basis.

Major signs of an endocrine disturbance are an inability to lose weight no matter what you do, infections that take a long time to heal, inflammation, and chronic fatigue. One or more glands may be out of balance—perhaps only the thyroid, maybe the adrenals too, or another combination. You'll have to figure out which ones are affected to know which supplements are appropriate to restore them. Whether you choose to focus your treatment or to support all of your glands at once, you need to monitor the effectiveness of your therapy.

One way to assess your hormonal situation is to have your physician do a hormone blood panel. But blood hormone levels can change frequently and dramatically with stress and other factors, and you can't get blood work done daily or weekly. That's why I recommend the self-monitoring system in my book *ProMetabolics: Your Personal Guide to Transformational Health and Healing (Designs for Wellness Press, Carlsbad, CA, 2008).* You can use it daily, weekly, and monthly to check your hormonal status and evaluate the effects of supplements, detox programs, and dietary modifications. I strongly suggest using my monitoring system to know what's going on and what's working for you.

Combining Therapies for Hormonal Issues

I've seen too many people taking four or five medications for what ails them, and then throwing in some vitamin C too. Maybe we need to turn it around, and use one drug with four or five nutritional supplements! When it's your body and your health, it's your call. The key is to use whatever you need—all types of healers and therapies—to restore yourself to a healthy state. Every healing method has its place, or it wouldn't exist.

A skilled physician or practitioner will typically mix and match a combination of therapies to address endocrine issues. A good approach to hormonal balancing, and to healing in general, is to combine supplements on the energetic level—homeopathic formulas—with supplements on the physical level—nutritional and herbal products. It's the approach I believe in and have used with great success.

A word on hormone replacement. When you take a synthetic hormone, the gland that normally produces that hormone will stop producing it, because the body registers that it's already present in the bloodstream. If need be, use natural hormone replacement therapy (HRT) until your body can get back to producing its own hormones—but combine therapies as described below, by stimulating the glands with homeopathic formulas, ensuring that the proper nutrients are present, and enhancing digestion. It would be absurd to take a synthetic hormone without also improving your digestion and nutrient absorption. For more information on HRT, see *ProMetabolics.*

Your Personalized Endocrine Program

1. Begin with the Basics

I strongly recommend that you begin any endocrine program with these fundamental elements, detailed in chapter 3:

- Create Triad Healing formulas to support the hormone triad of circles V, II, and IV. Mix up the foods and herbs in your combinations—it's always good to use a variety.
- Detoxify with blood-cleansing herbs and a bowel cleanse. A liver/gallbladder cleanse may also be necessary—a month between cleanses is suggested.
- Keep foundational nutrition and digestive aids constant. In addition to a whole-food concentrate such as Juice Plus+®, consider a green drink with ingredients such as chlorella, spirulina, alfalfa grass, barley grass, and wheatgrass—I like Matrixx Cellular Food (www.matrixx.ca). Take your enzymes and probiotics throughout. Effective digestion is an aspect of healing that must never be ignored!

2. Select Your Supplements

To tailor your program with specific supplements to support the affected gland(s) or influence the hormone(s) of interest, use the Endocrine Support Chart at the end of this chapter. The three categories are: homeopathic formulas, great for rebuilding and stimulating glands; physical supplements, namely herbs, vitamins, minerals, amino acids, pregnenolone, and DHEA; and as a last resort, whole-glandular products. See the appendix for more details on these and other helpful supplements, available at health food stores and through various online vendors:

- A good homeopathic formula for all three "master controllers"—pituitary, pineal, and hypothalamus—is Pituitary Liquid from MHP (www.mhpvitamins.com); it's also suggested for supporting other glands.
- MHP's homeopathic Thyroid Liquid and Adrenal Liquid are good for thyroid and adrenal support, but read the label for contraindications such as hyperthyroidism.
- Adrenal Response is a good herbal adrenal formula from Innate Response (www.innateresponse.com).
- Herbal tinctures called Bach Flower Remedies can help with the emotional issues that often accompany hormonal disturbance—especially if more than one gland is involved and your hormones are all over the place. You can pick emotion-specific tinctures or the Rescue Remedy for overall emotional balance (www.bachcentre.com).
- Mucuna and acetyl-l-carnitine, described earlier in this chapter, can be used for hypothalamus support.
- The adrenals need B-vitamins, particularly pantothenic acid (B_5), for cellular energy production and the conversion of pregnenolone to adrenal hormones. Pantothenic acid deficiency can lead to adrenal insufficiency. The suggested daily dose is 250–500 milligrams alone or in a B-complex.
- Vitamin C is also essential in adrenal hormone production. The thyroid, pancreas, and testicles accumulate vitamin C at 10–50 times its level in the bloodstream, while the

adrenals and pituitary accumulate it at 100 times the blood level, indicating its importance in endocrine function. It's best taken in buffered form combined with bioflavonoids.

- An iodine/iodide formula such as I-Throid from the Hall Center (www.thehallcenter.com) is suggested for the thyroid, because the body utilizes both mineral forms.
- You may wish to use a complete amino acid supplement—I use All-Basic from MHP. Tyrosine and tryptophan/5-HTP can be taken individually as indicated.
- Pregnenolone and DHEA, described earlier, are hormonal precursors, unlike whole-glandular formulas, which are extracts of animal glands and contain various substances including hormones. *Caution:* Only use a whole-glandular formula if you really truly need it. They're strong, and they may require professional supervision. They should be taken only five days a week for one to two months at most.

3. Monitor and Maintain

You're probably thinking, "This is a lot of stuff. Do I really have to take all these supplements?" Well, what did you expect? Your body's probably been in a toxic, deficient condition for years, and you have a real problem, especially if your health has deteriorated to a degenerative state. So the answer is yes. But will you have to stay on all these supplements forever? The answer is no. When you're healed and back in balance, you can maintain that balance with foundational nutrition.

Next, you're thinking, "How long do I have to be on this stuff?" It's generally best to evaluate your endocrine support program's effectiveness after working with it for two months. Then, when your self-monitoring or your physician's evaluation shows improvement and stability, you can begin to wean off the supplements; Pituitary Liquid is the last one to stop. You can, of course, stay on your Triad Healing foods as long as you'd like.

Every two months, get your hormonal status professionally monitored or monitor it yourself. To stay happy and healthy, continue with enzymes, probiotics, and a foundational whole-food concentrate for ongoing maintenance. And there you go!

Endocrine Program Examples

Hypothyroidism. Let's say you've learned that your thyroid function is low. First, you'd build your Triad Healing formulas, do a detoxification, and begin your foundational nutritional supplements and digestive aids. Next, you'd look at the thyroid row in the Endocrine Support Chart. You'd start with Pituitary Liquid, and then add Thyroid Liquid, I-Throid, and tyrosine. You might also want to take an all-purpose amino acid supplement. Then you'd monitor your condition. If two months on that regime didn't produce any change, you could add a thyroid glandular product and continue monitoring.

Hypoadrenalism. For low-functioning adrenals, you'd begin with your Triad Healing formulas, detox, foundational nutrition, and digestive aids. Next, you'd look at the adrenals row in the Endocrine Support Chart. You'd start with Pituitary Liquid, and then add Adrenal Response or Adrenal Liquid or both, along with pantothenic acid or a B-complex, and vitamin C. You might also want to take an all-purpose amino acid supplement. Then you'd monitor. If you experienced no change after two months, you could add DHEA or an adrenal glandular product—not both!—and continue monitoring.

Two glands out of balance. When two (or more) glands are imbalanced, you need a more intense program. A good suggestion in such a case would be to use pregnenolone as well as DHEA. As always, you'd begin with your Triad Healing formulas, detox, foundational nutrition, and digestive aids. If the imbalanced glands were the thyroid and adrenals, you'd then use DHEA and pregnenolone, Pituitary Liquid, Adrenal Response and/or Adrenal Liquid, I-Throid, tyrosine, pantothenic acid or a B-complex, vitamin C, and an all-purpose amino acid supplement. A program like that would support everything—and would also need to be monitored by a health practitioner.

ENDOCRINE SUPPORT CHART

GLAND/SITE	HORMONES/ NEUROTRANSMITTERS	SUPPLEMENTS
Pineal	Melatonin Serotonin	Pituitary Liquid Tryptophan/5-HTP Pregnenolone
Hypothalamus	Gonadotropin-releasing hormone (GnRH) Thyrotropin-releasing hormone (TSH) Acetylcholine Dopamine Serotonin	Pituitary Liquid Tyrosine Acetyl-l-carnitine Mucuna Pregnenolone
Pituitary	Adrenocorticotropic hormone (ACTH) Gonadotropins Growth hormone (GH) Prolactin Thyroid-stimulating hormone (TSH)	Pituitary Liquid Pituitary glandular Pregnenolone
Thyroid	Thyroxin (T4) Triiodothyronine (T3)	Pituitary Liquid Thyroid Liquid I-Throid Tyrosine Thyroid glandular
Adrenals	Adrenalin, noradrenalin Aldosterone Androstenedione Cortisone Dehydroepiandrosterone (DHEA) Estrogens, progesterone, testosterone	Pituitary Liquid Adrenal Response Adrenal Liquid Pantothenic acid/ B-complex Vitamin C DHEA Adrenal glandular

Chapter 7
Why Supplements Work—or Don't Work

Early in my practice, before I got into vibrational medicine, I believed that recommending the highest quality organic supplements to my clients was the best approach to healing. But I soon learned that ten people with the same illness or deficiency can be given the same nutrients from the same company—and they won't have the same results. One reason for this discrepancy is that an overloaded liver stressed with toxicity may not be able to process nutrients as well as another person's healthier liver. Supplement programs have to be individualized, as not everybody can respond to them the same way.

The body is always trying to keep itself in balance by acting and reacting metabolically. The body is not static, it is dynamic—down to the cellular level, it's constantly building up, breaking down, balancing, absorbing, and eliminating. When a toxin is taken in, the body neutralizes it and tries to restore balance. If the toxin exposure is prolonged, the body continually attempts to minimize its effect and may become deficient in an enzyme, mineral, or other important substance used in that process. What I didn't understand was that, in a similar fashion, the effects of a supplement can also be minimized in the body over time, and can lead to energy depletion.

Too Much of a Good Thing

You've probably experienced this: you start taking a super nutritional supplement, or herb, or medication, and you feel great for a short while—then it seems to stop working, and you don't feel the same. Why? In metabolizing the same substance over and over again, you can adapt to it, minimizing its effects over time and even depleting your energies in certain areas.

The body must be free to perform thousands of dynamic functions, rather than constantly responding to the one specific activity of the same substance. Maybe the body has healed itself at that level, and it's time to move on to something else, but it can't if you're still giving it the same treatment. The healing process stops, and the therapeutic effects can even be reversed, or other symptoms may appear as metabolizing the overused substance taxes your energy reserves.

This problem doesn't seem to occur, however, when the treatment is a variety of whole foods—only with strong herbs, some types of supplements, and medication. That's why traditional Chinese medicine uses an herbal remedy seasonally and for a specified duration, not indefinitely. And that's why a good practitioner changes a client's supplements and herbal programs every few months or more frequently. It's similar to athletic training: repeating the same exercise continually has limiting effects, whereas cross-training with different exercises promotes more balanced physical development rather than one area's over-development, and the body gets stronger overall.

Learning about this phenomenon was part of the basis for creating my Triad Healing approach, described in chapter 3. Rather than focusing exclusively on one problem or process, you're supporting and balancing all of the organs and meridians through the chosen triad while you're strengthening the body's weakest link. And by using a variety of foods and herbs in your therapeutic formulas, you're keeping the body on its toes.

Mass versus Energy: A Little Goes a Long Way

Consuming massive amounts of one food or nutrient isn't in synch with the human body's energies, and the resulting imbalance can cause a serious problem. You don't see many species of animals in the wild eating large amounts of the same food every day, and nothing else. The ape, for example, eats 117 different types of food—that's a lot of different energies. Your body, too, needs different foods, and in different amounts.

Natural foods are prepared by nature with low therapeutic "doses" of nutrients, so they can be "taken" on an ongoing basis. The technique of Kirlian photography has demonstrated that each food also has its own geometric energy structure, an individualized "energy signature." (Food processing and overcooking, unfortunately, often distorts or destroys that structure.) Nature is showing us that we can do more with less, because our cells recognize natural foods: the whole-food energy signatures match our cellular energy signatures. In quantum physics, this is called the law of resonance.

Energetic signatures are another part of the basis for Triad Healing. Certain groups of foods affect specific organs because of their particular energy signatures as well as their particular nutrient contents. The Triad Healing formulas use a variety of foods and herbs, matching their energies to the organs and meridians. They're in synch with nature, as natural food is nature's signature—and variety is the spice of life!

Whole Foods and Whole-Food Supplements

Over the last decade, the health industry has moved away from the megadose approach, as we've learned that small amounts of synergistic nutrients have a greater and more expansive effect on the body than massive amounts of single nutrients. Large amounts of single nutrients should only be intelligently used with professional advice and supervision. Nowadays, small amounts of vitamins and minerals are often mixed with whole-food concentrates, which have proven to be more readily absorbed and utilized by the body.

Whole foods contain a variety of departmentalized nutrients, known and unknown, that affect specific organs and support certain functions. Together, these nutrients act synergistically to benefit the body's systems. More than 15,000 phytochemicals were recently found in a single whole food. I wonder what we'll find in the future... Meanwhile, it's best to eat whole organic foods now, so we don't have to worry that we're not getting whatever vital compound we'll discover next.

I'm not saying we don't need supplements—we do, because our diets are typically lacking. Who really manages to eat 9–13 fruits and vegetables every day? Most people are too busy to make sure their diet includes all the different foods the body needs. But we should take our supplemental vitamins and minerals along with eating a variety of whole foods for better nutrient absorption and balance. And we can all use whole-food concentrates—vegetable, fruit, and especially berry—as a foundational, preventative nutritional support system.

Supplement Awareness and Professional Help

The greatest gift you can give to yourself—or somebody else—is knowledge about how to be healthy. Knowledge gives you power over disease. If you are reading up on nutrition and going out to buy supplements, be aware. Start off with whole-food supplements that are well-researched, and read about them. Consult a professional who uses supplementation, and get the right nutrients that you truly need. Otherwise, you end up wasting money on unnecessary supplements or buying things that may even cause you problems. Getting the proper advice is cheaper and more specific, and can save a lot of time and grief.

Important questions: Do you know what you're taking and why? Do you know the proper dose and how long to take it? Are the products from a reputable company? Do they have legitimate, primary research behind them? Are you absorbing what you're taking? Do you need to do a detoxification so your supplements will work better? People who work in the fields of nutrition and natural healing can answer these questions. You'll also find it helpful to evaluate the effects of your supplements by using the self-monitoring system described in my book *ProMetabolics: Your Personal Guide to Transformational Health and Healing (Designs for Wellness Press, Carlsbad, CA, 92008).*

Conclusion

No food, supplement, or drug heals the body. Your body speaks, your body heals. Your job is to create the conditions necessary for optimal health and healing, and to supply the necessary materials to the intelligence within. I hope that this book has expanded your understanding of the causes of acute and chronic ailments, motivated you to take charge of improving your health, and given you the information and tools to do that through detoxification and nutritional support. The fact is, your health is your responsibility, and your top priority.

What did I just say? Well, how can you take care of your children, or anyone or anything else, if you're sick and tired? Do you want to become a burden to someone by aging rapidly and developing a chronic condition? I personally want to live long enough to contribute my knowledge and expertise to society, and to accumulate some wealth to leave to my children. I'm sure you feel similarly. The greatest gift is life itself, and giving back to life is primary for our happiness. We're all together in this.

Stay Well,
Dr. Smokey Santillo

Appendix:
Get Smart Supplements

Here is a brief summary of some of the supplements discussed in this book, along with others that you can research if you're interested, plus some references for further reading. It's good to start with the suggested dose on the product's labeling; if needed, increase or decrease under professional guidance. Many books specify doses for certain conditions. *Note:* When you're working on endocrine support and hormonal balancing, a little can go a long way, because the energy of homeopathic formulas can increase the activity of other supplements.

Foundational Supplements

Digestive enzymes. Benefit virtually everyone. Take supplement containing all four major groups: amylase, protease, lipase, and cellulase. See chapters 3 and 5; see also proteolytic enzymes, below.

Juice Plus+®. Reduces oxidative stress. Supports immune system. Positively affects key indicators of cardiovascular wellness. Use for circulatory diseases and heart and blood vessel health. See chapters 3, 4, and 5.

Probiotics. "Friendly" intestinal bacteria. Vital digestive aid. Used for candida or other fungal problems. *Lactobacillus acidophilus* and *Bifidobacterium bifidum* are most used and most researched. Destroyed by antibiotics, take supplement to replenish. Dairy versions are suggested. See chapter 3.

Basic Nutrients and Phytonutrients

Amino acids. Building blocks of proteins, hormones, neurotransmitters, and more. Take all-purpose combination including essential amino acids: isoleucine, lysine, leucine, methionine, phenylalanine, threonine, tryptophan, and valine. Do not use single amino acids for longer than two months.

Suggested: All-Basic from MHP, www.mhpvitamins.com. See chapter 6; for much more information, see *ProMetabolics*.

Beta-carotene and mixed carotenoids. Precursors of vitamin A. Strong antioxidants. Deficiency linked to cataracts, skin diseases, and cancer. Food sources include apricot, beet, carrot, all greens, parsley, peach, and spinach. See chapters 4 and 5.

Essential fatty acids (EFAs). Crucial building blocks for nerve cells and cell membranes. Inhibit inflammation including arthritis, high blood pressure, and cardiovascular disease. If deficient, replaced in cell membranes by saturated fats, reducing oxygen and nutrient uptake and promoting aging. Most people don't get enough EFAs. Take supplement containing omega 3, 6, and 9 fatty acids. Suggested: Omega Nutrition's Essential Balance 3-6-9, made from organic flaxseed, pumpkin seed, sunflower, and organic unrefined olive oil; available through MHP, www.mhpvitamins.com.

Lycopene. Reddish pigment in tomatoes. Deposited in specific tissues, e.g., prostate gland. Helps prevent prostate cancer and heart disease. Helps prevent atherosclerosis by inhibiting cholesterol in low-density lipoproteins (LDLs) from oxidizing and forming plaque on artery walls.

Vitamin C and bioflavonoids. Antioxidants and powerful anti-inflammatories. Food sources include berries, other fruits, and grape seed and grape skin extracts. See chapters 5 and 6.

Herbs

Ashwagandha (winter cherry, Indian ginseng). Used in Ayurvedic medicine as aphrodisiac and diuretic, also for memory loss. In formulas for energy and sexual vitality. Useful to men and women for rejuvenating bones, muscles, adrenal glands, reproductive system, and other tissues.

Cayenne (capsicum). Hot red pepper unequalled at normalizing circulation. Used for arteriosclerosis, arthritis, fever, frostbite, gastrointestinal disorders, muscle pain, and rheumatic conditions. Excellent for mucus conditions, congestion, and detoxification. Potentiates effects of other herbs. Use daily in food or ¼ teaspoon in water as circulatory tonic. See chapter 3.

Ginkgo biloba. Improves circulation, particularly to brain. Counteracts free radicals. Strengthens capillaries. Extract approved in Europe for Alzheimer's disease. See chapter 3.

Mucuna. Reported nerve tonic and mild aphrodisiac. Influences mood and sexuality. Supports libido in aging individuals. Active constituents include antioxidants and dopamine precursor l-dopa. Used in India for Parkinson's disease, under study as long-term treatment. See chapter 6.

More Detoxification, Antioxidant, Anti-Infection, and Anti-Inflammatory Agents

Alpha-lipoic acid. "Antioxidant workhorse." Protects cell membranes. Good for athletes. Helps eliminate heavy metals; for mercury toxicity, take 300–600 milligrams daily. Used for tingling hands and feet from diabetic neuropathy. Stimulates eyes' production of glutathione (see below), protecting against cataracts. Recycles/regenerates vitamins C and E and coenzyme Q10 (see below). Take with meals.

Coenzyme Q10 (CoQ10, ubiquinone). Potent antioxidant. Believed essential for human life. Beneficial for heart, brain, and gums. Important in adenosine triphosphate (ATP) synthesis, stimulating cellular metabolic processes. Regulates oxidation of fats and sugars into cellular energy. Elevates energy and extends cell life. Strengthens capillaries and normalizes blood pressure. Boosts immune system capabilities. Vital role in prevention and treatment of many major diseases. Like vitamin E, protects cell membrane phospholipids. Production decreases 50 percent from young adulthood; deficiency causes fatigue. See chapter 5.

Glutathione. Compound of amino acids cysteine, glutamic acid, and glycine. Antioxidant acting outside cells. Effective in heavy metal detoxification. Helps liver detoxify carcinogens and protects it from alcohol damage. Used for variety of diseases. Suggested dose 500 milligrams daily, with other antioxidants. Food sources include acorn squash, asparagus, avocado, broccoli, cantaloupe, grapefruit, okra, orange, peach, potato, spinach, strawberry, tomato, watermelon, and zucchini.

Methionine. Antioxidant, sulfur-containing essential amino acid. Source of methyl molecules, used in RNA and DNA synthesis and binding free radicals. Aids brain's production of neurotransmitters and phospholipids. With lysine, converted to l-carnitine and acetyl-l-carnitine (see below). Converted to s-adenosyl methionine (see below); both used for depression, suicidal tendency, and mental sluggishness. Converted to amino acid cysteine; both powerful in heavy metal detoxification. (*Note:* Buildup of conversion compound homocysteine can increase risk of heart attack and stroke if deficient in folic acid, B_6, and B_{12}; take B-vitamins if high homocysteine.) Suggested dose 800–3,000 milligrams daily. Food sources include beef, chicken, lentil, liver, pumpkin seed, and sardine. See chapter 6.

Methyl sulfonyl methane (MSM). Non-metallic sulfur compound; sulfur important in connective tissue formation, joints, hair, skin, nails, organs, blood, and insulin. Used for joint degeneration and inflammation. Reduces lactic acid buildup. Helps with allergy, arthritis, asthma, calcium deposits, circulation, gum disease, lupus, pain, scar tissue, sinus infection, stiffness, swelling, and hyperacidity of stomach and intestines. Suggested dose 2–20 grams daily for less than two weeks, professionally monitored. *(Jacob S, Lawrence R. The Miracle of MSM: The Natural Solution for Pain. GP Putnam's Sons, NY, 1999)*

Proteolytic enzymes (proteases). Include pancreatic proteases chymotrypsin and trypsin, bromelain from pineapple, papain from papaya, and fungal proteases. Break proteins into amino acids. Help immune system by breaking down antigen-antibody complexes in infection and autoimmune disease. History of use for arthritis, cancer, circulatory problems, fibromyalgia, infection, inflammation, lupus, pain, sports injuries, and swelling. Very useful after tooth extraction and surgery. Take immediately for colds, fever, and respiratory or sinus mucus conditions. See chapter 5.

Hormones and Hormone Support

Adrenal Response. Herbal adrenal support. From Innate Response, www.innateresponse.com. See chapter 6.

Dehydroepiandrosterone (DHEA). Precursor of steroids including sex hormones. Synthesized from pregnenolone (see below). Declines around age 40–45. Increases acetylcholine. Strengthens sexual health. Improves neurological function, mood, stress disorders, and immune function. Can help normalize hormone levels. Can restore hypo-functioning adrenals and counteract progression of inflammatory diseases such as rheumatoid arthritis. Elevates insulin-like growth factor, potentially counteracting fat accumulation and neurological problems of aging. See chapters 5 and 6.

I-Throid. Iodine/iodide formula for thyroid support. From The Hall Center, www.thehallcenter.com. See chapter 6.

Melatonin. Neurohormone synthesized from serotonin and secreted during darkness. Great relaxer, used for insomnia, also effective against jet lag. Immunostimulant, helps control infections and cancer. Decline results in loss of hormone synchronization and sleep loss, potentially starting chain of pathological aging-associated processes. See chapter 6.

Pituitary Liquid. Homeopathic support for endocrine system, specifically pituitary, pineal, and hypothalamus. Use for all hormonal imbalances. From MHP, www.mhpvitamins.com. See chapter 6.

Pregnenolone. Prohormone synthesized from cholesterol. Ultimate precursor for entire family of steroid hormones. Excellent candidate for hormone precursor therapy of endocrine disorders. "The compound possesses—at least in traces—every independent main pharmacological action which has hitherto been shown to be exhibited by any steroid hormone." See chapter 6. *(Roberts E. Pregnenolone—from Selye to Alzheimer and a model of the pregnenolone sulfate binding site on the GABA$_A$ receptor. Biochem Pharmacol 1995 49:1–16)*

Thyroid Liquid. Homeopathic support for thyroid. Helps in hypothyroid conditions. *Note:* Do not use in hyperthyroidism. From MHP, www.mhpvitamins.com. See chapter 6.

Whole-glandular formulas. Combination extracts derived from animal glands, can contain hormones and other stimulating substances. For adrenal, thyroid, and/or pituitary support. Use only if necessary after first trying other endocrine therapies, e.g., homeopathic and herbal. Take for only one to two months, with professional monitoring. See chapter 6.

Brain and Neurotransmitter Support

Acetyl-l-carnitine. Derivative of l-carnitine or amino acids lysine and methionine. Maintains brain's metabolism of acetylcholine. Involved in sexuality. Improves dopamine levels and prevents significant amount of aging-associated brain cell loss. Studies show improvement in dementia. See chapter 6.

Choline and lecithin. Precursors to acetylcholine. Most commonly used memory-enhancing nutrients. Choline also critical constituent of fat in brain cell membranes.

Gamma amino-butyric acid (GABA). Amino acid acting as neurotransmitter throughout nervous system and brain. By filling brain receptor sites, slows or blocks excitatory messages and inhibits rapid-firing nerve responses, relaxing muscles and mind. Good for mood disorders, plays major role in inhibiting anxiety and panic. Usually taken as 500-milligram capsule dissolved in water three times daily. Dose half-hour before bedtime promotes relaxation and sleep. Taken with magnesium and amino acids glutamine, taurine, and glycine. Food sources include fish and wheat bran. *(Ricketts M. The Great Anxiety Escape. Matulungin Publishing, La Mesa, CA, 1990)*

Phosphatidylserine. Important phospholipid (phosphorus-fat combination) in brain. Contributes to cell membrane integrity and fluidity. Helps neurotransmitter release and nutrient transport. Used in elderly patients for depression and impaired mental function, mood, and behavior. Synthesis requires essential fatty acids (see above).

S-adenosyl methionine (SAMe). Form of methionine (see above). Increases conversion of l-dopa to serotonin and dopamine. Antidepressant in most individuals. Start with 200 milligrams twice daily and increase to 400 milligrams three times daily. *Caution:* Do not take SAMe if you have bipolar disorder, as this has resulted in serious negative outcomes of anxiety and panic. *(Rogers SA. Depression: Cured at Last! Sand Key Publishing, Sarasota, FL, 1997)*

Tryptophan. Essential amino acid, serotonin precursor (see also 5-hydroxytryptophan, below). Food sources include banana, brown rice, chickpea, chocolate, cottage cheese, date, egg, fish, mango, milk, oat, peanut, poultry, pumpkin seed, red meat, sesame, spirulina, sunflower, and yogurt. See chapter 6.

5-hydroxytryptophan (5-HTP). Form of tryptophan (see above) that crosses blood brain barrier more effectively. Precursor for serotonin synthesis. Human and animal studies indicate utility for range of health problems including alcoholism, anxiety, depression, eating disorders, insomnia, panic attacks, and premenstrual syndrome. See chapter 6.

Index

— Notes —

— Notes —

ORDER FORM

Name: ______________________________

Address: ______________________________

____

Phone: ______________________________

Email Address: ______________________________

	Quantity	Price	Total
Your Body Speaks…	_____	12.95	_____
ProMetabolics	_____	29.95	_____
Natural Healing with Herbs	_____	16.95	_____
Food Enzymes	_____	9.95	_____

TOTAL ______________

Mail: Vartabedian & Associates, P.O. Box 1671, Carlsbad, CA 92018
Fax: 760-804-5996
Phone: 888-796-5229
Online: www.SmokeySantillo.com

Card #: ______________________________ Exp.: ________

✓ one: ❑ MC ❑ VISA ❑ AMEX ❑ Discover CVV2: ________

Signature: ______________________________

ORDER FORM

Name: ______________________________

Address: ______________________________

____

Phone: ______________________________

Email Address: ______________________________

	Quantity	Price	Total
Your Body Speaks...	_____	12.95	_____
ProMetabolics	_____	29.95	_____
Natural Healing with Herbs	_____	16.95	_____
Food Enzymes	_____	9.95	_____

TOTAL ______________

Mail: Vartabedian & Associates, P.O. Box 1671, Carlsbad, CA 92018
Fax: 760-804-5996
Phone: 888-796-5229
Online: www.SmokeySantillo.com

Card #: ______________________________ Exp.: _______

✓ one: ❑ MC ❑ VISA ❑ AMEX ❑ Discover CVV2: _______

Signature: ______________________________